LEARNING TO LIVE AGAIN

LEARNING
TO
LIVE
AGAIN

MY TRIUMPH OVER CANCER

Joel Solkoff

Holt, Rinehart and Winston
New York

Published by Holt, Rinehart and Winston,
383 Madison Avenue, New York, New York 10017

Published simultaneously in Canada by Holt, Rinehart and
Winston of Canada, Limited.

Library of Congress Cataloging in Publication Data

Solkoff, Joel.
Learning to Live Again.
1. Hodgkin's disease—United States—Biography.
2. Solkoff, Joel.   I. Title.
RC644.S57   1983   362.1′9699446′0924 [B] 82-18743
ISBN 0-03-057647-4

First Edition

Designer: Joy Taylor
Printed in the United States of America
1   3   5   7   9   10   8   6   4   2

ISBN 0-03-057647-4

This book is lovingly dedicated to my wife Diana.

"Do you know what I have come for?" says Jurgen, blustering and splendid in his glittering shirt and gleaming armor. "For I warn you I am justice."

"I think you are lying, and I am sure you are making an unnecessary noise. In any event, justice is a word, and I control all words."

—James Branch Cabell
Jurgen, A Comedy of Justice

LEARNING TO LIVE AGAIN

1

I DO NOT HAVE CANCER ANYMORE. The disease was treated by conventional radiation therapy, and my physicians say that it has been eradicated. I believe that I have been cured, despite a recurring nightmare that a doctor is examining my body, checking for lumps.

Today, I had lunch with Laura in the oak-paneled dining room of the Hay-Adams Hotel. We each had two drinks and needed more. Our love affair became a casualty of the cancer cure. Too much intensity was confined to too short a period of time, time that always seemed to be running out. Although we tried afterward, we were unable to salvage our relationship. Today, I told Laura that I am engaged to marry another woman—Diana, whom I met after the cancer experience was over. Laura and I toasted to the future—a future that we will not share.

It is spring here in Washington. The cherry blossoms are

out early. Spring this year feels the same as it did five years ago. I continue to live in the same city and in the same apartment. At thirty-three, I am too young to write my memoirs. Yet that is what I am doing, reliving the period five years ago when I was diagnosed as having cancer and feared death. The diagnosis and its treatment—over a period of six months—was the worst experience of my life. Remembering how poorly I behaved is worse than remembering the physical pain and the fear.

Now, five years later, my statistical category has changed. Today I conform to the American Cancer Society's definition of cured: five years without a recurrence of symptoms. A generation ago my type of cancer, Hodgkin's disease, was described as "invariably fatal." A generation ago I could not have survived five years. I would not have lived to interview family, friends, and physicians, nor to revisit the hospital in which I was operated upon and treated. The difficulties of remembering and surviving would have been denied me.

ON FRIDAY AFTERNOON, April 23, 1976, I am sitting in a doctor's office worrying. Worrying is something that I do a lot and am good at. At the time I do not realize that I have much more reason for concern than when I normally worry about (a) money, (b) getting the article in on time, (c) my relationship with Laura, (d) finishing the book, (e) cleaning the apartment, and so on. Specifically, I am in the waiting room of Aaron Falk's * office because there is a small lump—about the size of a golf ball—under my right arm. The lump does not hurt, and

* While all characters in this book are real, several names have been changed.

it is noticeable to no one but me. However, it has been there for a number of weeks, and several times a day I find myself feeling under my armpit to check whether it has gone away. The lump has joined my mental list of things to worry about.

Given how regularly I worry about my health—running to a doctor's office at the first sign of a cold, a sore throat, or a backache—I do not anticipate that my first appointment with Dr. Falk will be noticeably different from previous appointments with other doctors. My experience as a mild hypochondriac is that doctors find my ailments boring. I leave their offices feeling embarrassed for bothering them and stupid for paying so much money to find out that there's nothing wrong with me.

Indeed, I have made the appointment because I want to be reassured that nothing is wrong with me. This time I am sufficiently concerned about the lump that I am willing to risk the likely embarrassment and expense. However, the longer I sit in the waiting room, the more convinced I become that the lump is inconsequential and that it will probably disappear if I wait long enough. I am convinced that Dr. Falk, whom I have yet to meet, will be polite, but in a tone that will imply that doctors go to medical school to cure really sick people and why does he have to waste his time seeing obviously healthy people like me.

As I read the plastic sign welcoming patients to talk about physician fees with the physician, I decide that now that I am in the doctor's office, I can stop worrying about the lump and start worrying about money. My concern about money at this time has a rational aspect to it. As a free-lance writer my income is precarious. I have difficulty obtaining insurance. My previous policy, with Stan, a friend of a friend who agreed to let me join his group plan, was terminated because Stan pocketed the payments rather than sending them to Blue Cross. That experience has made me feel insecure about my current plan, with the newly formed Washington Independent Writers. The paperwork is already fouled up. Despite the organization's reassurance that my membership card has been processed and is in the mail, I worry that I may not be covered by insurance at all. So as I appraise the doctor's office, which is in an expensive neighborhood, provides free parking for its patients, has its own laboratory on the premises, and offers a spacious waiting room (where a large potted plant has cedar chips covering the soil), I am concerned that the tests and doctor's fee will be more than I can afford—and all for a complaint that will probably turn out to be nothing.

Aaron Falk begins, as doctors do, by asking why I have come to see him. I tell him about the lump under my arm, that it has been there for several weeks, that it doesn't hurt, and that it hasn't gone away. I ask, "Is it serious?"

He says, "I don't know yet. First let's get the usual questions out of the way. Then we'll go next door where you'll take your clothes off and I'll examine you. We'll take some routine blood tests and a chest X ray. When we're done with that we'll come back here and I'll tell you what I think, assuming I think anything. Okay? Now, how old are you?"

"Twenty-eight."

"Profession?"

"I'm a writer, specializing in agricultural policy." We talk about that for a while.

We get along instantly. Our ability to communicate seems uncanny. There are not the usual barriers that separate doctor from patient. Dr. Falk is only seven years older than I, so we relate as peers. He is not condescending toward me, as are physicians who make themselves inaccessible because of their specialized knowledge.

BY THE END of the day, I was calling him by his first name, because it seemed artificial for him to call me Joel while I was calling him Dr. Falk. In retrospect, I must have decided to trust Aaron as soon as we met, when I entered his private office and sat down on the wood-and-wicker chair.

At the time of this first visit, I knew nothing about his educational background. Dr. Falk graduated from Harvard College and went to the University of Pennsylvania Medical School. I also did not find out, until much later, that Dr. Falk and I shared a similar religious upbringing: he attended the Hebrew Academy of Washington; I went to the Hebrew Academy of Miami Beach. While I soon rejected the ritual and ever-present discipline of orthodox Judaism, Dr. Falk continued to observe it. Indeed given the additional distance I was then putting between myself and Judaism, if I had known about our shared religious background, it would have put distance between us.

AARON is the same height as I am—5 feet 10 inches. He is thin and although prematurely gray, he looks younger than he is. Our preliminary small talk clearly makes him impatient, an impatience he has difficulty curbing. He recognizes the necessity of getting acquainted, but fidgets as he sits, uncertain about what to do with his large hands and arms, patently restraining the impulse to dash down the corridor and "do something." This impatient, almost distracted manner extends to his dress. He is wearing a regulation jacket and tie, but it is that and no more, he looks neither dapper nor even coordinated, his clothes the expression of a man who has more important concerns. He talks in spurts, the way professors do who are more comfortable with scholarship than students. Sentences are strung together rapid-fire, followed by long pauses while he weighs each word. He suspects that he's transparent and that everyone knows what he's thinking when he's thinking it. So Aaron smiles a lot during his embarrassed pauses or when I am talking too long, as if to say, *Dealing with people comes awkwardly, but I want you to like me.* The smiles work. His eyes light up, expressing interest, even tenderness.

"Marital status?" Aaron asks.

I must be more frightened than I realize. Rather than say, "Single and divorced," which is how I usually automatically answer the question, I launch into an exposition on the intricacies of New York State's divorce laws, which five years previous made it more convenient to get an annulment than a divorce. When I respond to a simple question with a long, irrelevant answer, it means that I don't want to deal with whatever's going on.

On the way to the examination room he asks how I've been referred to him. I say, "I see Dr. Bernstein" (an ear-nose-and-throat specialist whom I visit for colds and allergy attacks). "I asked the secretary what kind of doctor specializes in lumps. She said an internist and gave me your name."

"You certainly are lucky," Aaron says. "Not only am I an internist, but this office's specialty is hematology." (He does not mention that the office's other specialty is oncology—the treatment of cancer.)

We are now inside the examination room and he says, "Take off your clothes and I'll be right back."

"What's hematology?"

He stops moving and answers. "It deals with disorders of the blood. It means, you might say, that lumps are our bag."

What he says frightens me. Instead of asking the obvious—"Do I have a disorder of the blood?"—I revert to worrying about money. Telling him of my concern I say, "Tests are expensive and I'm short of funds right now. Can you go easy on the tests?"

Abruptly, he places his right arm against the door, as if to stop himself from exiting. Turning toward me, he seems suddenly angry as he says, "Nobody's going to tell me how to practice medicine. If I order tests, it's because I think they're necessary. I'm a doctor and my concern is your health. I don't give a damn about the money. If you can't afford it, then you can't afford it. We'll work something out. You'll pay me if you can, and if you can't then you can't. Money is the last thing we need to worry about now. I'm not going to let you tie my hands by telling me not to order the tests I need to practice quality medicine."

After I take off my clothes, he feels the lump under my right arm, asking whether it hurts as he touches it. It doesn't hurt. Kneading my skin with his fingertips, he feels for lumps under my left arm, under my ears and behind my neck, across my abdomen, and at my groin. There aren't any other lumps.

He asks, "Do you have sudden chills or wake up sweating in the middle of the night?

"Have you been running a fever?

"Do you have sudden outbreaks of itching?

"Have you recently experienced sudden and unexplained weight loss?

"Do you suffer from loss of appetite?"

I answer no to all the questions, and when they stop, I say, "Why are you asking me this? What's wrong with me?"

He says, "I don't know that anything's wrong with you. Go to the lab around the corner—he points the way—"and they'll take some blood. The nurse there will direct you to the X-ray room. After you're done with the chest X ray, get dressed and return to my office. Then, we'll talk."

If there were more room in the office, he'd probably pace, trying to figure out some way of saying what he wants to say without frightening me. Instead, he leans awkwardly against a bookshelf and, in a rush to get it over with, blurts out, "Look, I don't know what the lump is. It's probably nothing, but I don't know. I think it's a good idea for you to see a surgeon so he can remove the lump from your arm and we can examine it and find out what it is." He is trying hard to convey as much information as possible, so I can understand his perspective and make a rational decision. He smiles abruptly, as if to apologize for what he's just told me, and asks, "Are you willing to see a surgeon?"

"I guess so."

"Can you do it right now?"

"Yes."

He gets on the phone and calls a surgeon named Cory Simpson and inquires whether he can see me right away. He can. Aaron says about me, "Yes, he's perfectly capable of walking over. In fact, I'll tell him to run over. He'll be there in a few minutes."

Aaron gives me Simpson's address, which is about five blocks away. He says, "Look, it's Friday afternoon and you're lucky that Dr. Simpson can see you right now. I want him to have a look at your arm. Then come back here so we can talk."

As I leave his office, he calls after me. "Hey, there's nothing to worry about. I don't want you to be alarmed. It's best to do these things quickly, just to be on the safe side."

As I am crossing L Street and New Hampshire Avenue, it does not occur to me to question why I am listening to this doctor's urgent instructions or why I trust him. I am puzzled because never before has a physician taken my physical ailments quite this seriously. Fear is creeping up on me, fear because the doctor has asked me specific questions and because it seems that I have a specific disease; fear because he says he specializes in disorders of the blood and by implication that's what I may have; fear because I am en route to a surgeon. I have never had an operation, and I'm a coward when it comes to pain. Fear because a doctor thinks that an operation is necessary at all. But I don't actually *feel* frightened yet. I can tell that the fear is coming, but am able to put it off, not wanting to be afraid, too busy concentrating on getting to Simpson's office and on obtaining as quickly as possible a new range of information that I'll need to deal with this situation. I know that I'll be frightened later, but for the moment my curiosity is stronger than the fear. I consciously decide—like Dr. Spock in "Star Trek"—to banish my emotions and concentrate on being logical.

I arrive at Dr. Simpson's office and am filling out the insurance form when the doctor comes out. "Are you Mr. Solkoff?" Pointing to the insurance form, he says, "You can do that later. Why don't you come into my office?"

Simpson is also not much older than I. He is tall, thin, and wears a tapered three-piece designer suit. Among George Washington University medical students, who are notoriously hard on their instructors, he has a reputation for being a very fast and very good surgeon. Right away, I find him to be unpretentious and easy to understand. He feels the lump under my arm and says that he doesn't think there will be any problem removing it. He reassures me that the operation won't be painful (which I don't believe), that I'll be awake while he does it, and that I can return to work right away.

I say, "What's the rush? Why did Dr. Falk tell me to run over here?"

"Aaron has a tendency to be enthusiastic. He probably thinks it's a good idea to find out quickly what that 'lump,' as you call it, really is."

"What do you think it is?"

"I don't know. You'll have to ask Aaron."

SIMPSON'S ATTITUDE toward me, from the beginning, was matter-of-fact. Later, he told me, "In reality, as a surgeon I was actually put in the position of being just a technician. I was not making major decisions regarding your care. The major decisions were really made by Dr. Falk—and you, of course." He explained that surgeons, like anyone else, would prefer to be creative and in a position of authority.

Instead, as often happens, he was asked to do a routine task which he had done hundreds of times before. He was perfectly willing to explain the procedure to me and consistently answered every question asked about surgery and possible complications. However, regarding speculations on my diagnosis and life chances he continually referred me back to Aaron, whom he regarded as my primary physician. Whenever I asked whether he thought a procedure Aaron recommended was necessary, he said yes, telling me that Aaron was a respected physician who specialized in conditions like mine and whose judgment was trustworthy. Eventually Simpson told me, "You and I are relatively close in age, and since I could avoid thinking about your dying, I did."

Simpson and I never became friends, as opposed to my relationship with Aaron. I still don't know Simpson well, and I doubt that many people do. Yet I respected him. He was easy to be with during painful and stressful situations. Like Aaron, he has an off-beat sense of humor, which we shared and enjoyed, and while there was nothing memorable about our jokes and bantering, it made future events easier that we all "horsed around" (as Aaron put it), often in a self-deprecating way. Given the closeness in our ages, none of us took offense or felt threatened when I complained about Simpson's sutures or Aaron's plans for treatment or when they complained about my behavior. Had they been much older, or had I been much older, my relationship with my doctors would have been more decorous—making the whole experience grimmer.

BACK AT AARON'S OFFICE, I ask what he thinks the lump is. He says, "It may be nothing at all, just some fatty tissue."

"But you think it's something else?"

"I don't think it's something else. I don't know what it is. That's why I want to find out."

"What else might it be?"

"It's probably a benign tumor."

I am frightened by the word *tumor*. Having assumed that I'd never have to deal with a tumor, each time the word appears in conversation I tune it out. "If it's benign, why is it swollen?" I ask Aaron.

"All tumors are enlargements, abnormal growths. Most just happen, for reasons which are complicated and about which we're not entirely sure. Most tumors are benign, which means they're not serious, and when we remove them, there's nothing to worry about. The chances are that yours is benign and that when Dr. Simpson removes it, you and I will be done and you can go about your business."

"And if it's a serious tumor?" I don't want to say the word *cancer*.

"I don't think it's serious, but if it is, then we'll cross that bridge when we come to it."

We talk about scheduling for the operation. He wants the tumor out of me as quickly as possible. I realize that walking around worrying that I have "something serious" when I probably don't is stupid, and the sooner I know the better. But I don't want someone else or something else controlling my life. I have an article to complete on Cesar Chavez, which Marty Peretz, the owner of *The New Republic*, commissioned and is expecting. Already, I am beginning the process of negotiating, trying to fit the problem of my tumor into my schedule. Aaron says firmly, "Don't wait too long. This is something that should be taken care of right away." I promise to call Simpson's office and schedule an appointment.

$$\boxed{2}$$

ITIS LATE Friday afternoon and I am scared. I need a drink badly. I need a friend. I need Laura. I call her and we meet at a bar at Nineteenth and K called The Owl and the Pussycat. She has a whiskey sour and I have a Scotch on the rocks.

YEARS LATER, Laura said, "Are you ever going to get me out of your system?" It was a rhetorical question, the kind one asks when too many events have passed to make an answer possible. In this case, however, the answer is that I will never get her out of my system. I will always love her in a way that makes my heart beat faster and my palms sweat. Some people—either by accident or fate—enter our lives and we are forever different. For me, Laura remains one of those people. We never could learn how to live together, but we will always love each other. It is, of course, impossible to describe such a relationship. Most who experience it have the good sense not to try. On that day in late April, as we sat in that poorly lit bar with cheap red tablecloths, our love affair was at its most intense period and, as it would turn out, its most fragile.

LAURA TAUNTON SHELBY CONSTABLE. She is 5 feet 4½ inches tall and weighs 112 pounds. She has green eyes and shoulder-length dark-blond hair. She is beautiful in a way that defies classification. Her long angular face with its high cheekbones and rigid jaw causes strangers on the street to stare at her. Her figure is lean; her long legs graceful, and she dresses and frequently acts with a flamboyant carelessness, as if saying, "I don't care what men think of my looks."

But she cares intensely. An old boyfriend once called her Iron Jaw, and she remains sensitive to comments about her appearance. Often she is ready to rebuff remarks that never come. When we first met she wore blue jeans and dark turtlenecks, like a uniform. It was what she called her "tough-guy period." Recently she has begun to "soften her image," wearing cotton and silk blouses which reveal her braless breasts. The best restaurants in town have not yet adjusted to blue jeans, and each supper presents a new challenge to headwaiters to decline to seat her, a challenge she always wins. When she is alone, she goes off to spend hours in exclusive Georgetown boutiques, trying on outfits she rarely buys and never wears— imagining she is throwing a society party at which she devastates her guests with her looks and her wit.

YEARS LATER, trying to keep my reportorial objectivity, I interviewed her about what she thought in 1976.

"How did you feel about me?"

"I loved you."

"Why did you love me?"

"Because you were attractive and exciting and a young man on the rise, and because you treated me well."

"Wasn't I conceited?"

"Yes, and you were arrogant too."

"Wasn't I self-centered?"

"You've always been self-centered."

"Then why did you love me?"

"For the reasons I listed."

"Did you think we were going to get married?"

"Yes."

"Did you want to marry me?"

"Yes."

"Were you frightened about what might happen to me?"

"Yes."

"Why?"

"Listen, you idiot. I loved you. I cared what happened to you. I was worried that something might be wrong with you. I loved you and didn't want you hurt. I loved you and didn't want to lose you. I was scared and I was frightened and I was angry that something might happen to you. Does that answer your dumb questions?"

SHE WAS the most honest woman I'd ever met. I was used to manipulative women, who tried to control me and do so indirectly. I once married a woman like that. Laura was direct, often abrasively so. She was not interested in manipulating or controlling me, and she wouldn't put up with my periodic attempts to manipulate her. Sex with her was the most exciting thing either of us had ever known. There was passion, energy, screaming, and tenderness. We were funny together, sparring with each other verbally, getting drunk and laughing at jokes that only we understood. Even when we were sober, everything seemed funny in a cynical, offbeat way.

ABOUT A MONTH before that Friday afternoon, Laura got the final decree on a long and sticky divorce. She worked her way through five lawyers, trying to find one "mean and vicious enough" to deal with her husband. Now in the spring of 1976, after two years of waiting for the divorce, it looks as if we might finally live together and get married. There is, however, the lump under my right arm.

Early that morning I mentioned my lump for the first time and she had one of her frequent bursts of temper. "Don't you know that there are people dying of cancer around here all the time? What are you going to do, wait until your arm falls off before you see a doctor?" I calmed her down, saying that I had an appointment that afternoon. She apologized, telling me that her mother and her former husband always delayed medical attention until they manipulated her into pushing them to the doctor.

As we drink, I tell her what happened at Aaron's office. There is not much to say. We both know that further information awaits the outcome of the operation. We are both frightened, both intent on reassuring each other. It doesn't matter what we say. What matters is that we are together. I need to look at her, to know that she is with me. Holding her hand makes me feel less afraid.

WHEN I FINALLY schedule the operation it is for the following Friday. Simpson wants to do it more quickly, but I don't want my work week interrupted. It is a long seven days. I work on the Cesar Chavez article maniacally, as if my life were dependent upon its completion. I have to keep reminding myself to pay attention to my routine and avoid thinking about disease and death. Characteristically I do not consider what the wait is doing to me emotionally or how it is affecting Laura. Stubbornly I keep to my list of priorities. My work comes first. Only when I am done with this project will I allow myself the time to think about my feelings and Laura's feelings.

Laura drives me to George Washington University Hospital in her forest-green Volkswagen bug. Green is Laura's favorite color. She says that it matches her eyes and that it is the color of hope. The weather is beautiful—a rare Washington occurrence that happens during the brief spring and fall seasons. I don't know when most people prefer to have operations, but today the weather contributes to the feeling that I'd rather be doing something else. Having thought that surgical appointments were difficult to obtain, I am frightened that this one has been obtained so quickly and that Simpson has been so willing to accommodate my schedule.

Simpson suggested that I eat breakfast before the operation. That seemed peculiar, but he said it was a good idea not to feel weak. "After all," he joked, "I don't want you fainting on me." Perhaps it really didn't make any difference whether I ate or not, and Simpson was simply suggesting doing something routine to make me feel less anxious.

So first Laura and I drive to the elegant Hay-Adams Hotel, which is across Lafayette Park from the White House. Typical of my restaurant habits, the Hay-Adams is too expensive. Coffee is served from a silver pot, and croissants on heated plates. Both of us are too anxious to eat, and we pick at our food, trying to pretend that neither of us is worried. I ask trivial questions: "Would you like some more water? Would you like some more butter? Are you sure you don't want strawberries? Is the croissant hot enough for you?" She tells a string of one-line jokes about Jerry Ford's tripping and bumping into things. I don't want to talk about the coming operation, and Laura isn't going to mention it unless I do. Even though it is early morning, I want to order a Bloody Mary, but don't out of concern that alcohol will react adversely with the surgical drugs. We leave earlier than necessary. I am nervous about being late—or more accurately, I am nervous.

I am wearing a tie and jacket for my operation because I feel more prepared when I dress up. Since this is my first visit to George Washington University Hospital, the receptionist at the "In & Out" surgery room has to create a new file for me. Laura and I sit in the small waiting room while I fill out the form. There are other people, other couples. One woman is squeezing her husband's hand, her knuckles turning white. I try to reassure her with a smile, but she looks away. Another woman, sitting next to the magazine table, is crying quietly. On the form in the blank requesting "Closest Relative," I write *Laura Constable, friend.* I sign the form after reading "Dr. Simpson has explained to me the nature of the operation to be performed . . . and the possible risks and consequences associated with this type of operation or procedure, and the other risks that are attendant to the performance of any surgical procedure, and I do hereby voluntarily consent to said operation or procedure."

Earlier in the week, Laura suggested that she rearrange her schedule so she could wait for me during the operation. Laura has been working as an administrative assistant for the Migrant Legal Action Program (MLAP). We met at MLAP nearly two years previously when I was the organization's newsletter editor. Laura's job involves supporting the executive director, keeping the office's attorneys up-to-date on policy decisions, dividing up the secretaries' work load, ordering supplies, and making sure that everyone gets paid. At best it is a demanding job, and because the office—typical of many nonprofit organizations—is not run in a businesslike way, Laura has been trying to change jobs. She is frustrated by board members who meddle in day-to-day activities and undermine the new executive director, whose predecessor was forced to resign. Most staff attorneys have quit or have been fired within the previous two years; morale is low and egos are high. The organization, dependent on federal money, has been through so many funding crises that it seems normal for employees to wonder whether they'll get their next check. That morning the chairman of the board, who is a "superlawyer," a partner in one of Washington's largest and most prestigious firms, and MLAP's executive director are scheduled to meet with Laura to resolve some of the organization's problems. So I realize that Laura has other things to do besides be with me.

Anyway, I am intent on dealing by myself with whatever comes up. By nature I am afraid of showing my weaknesses to anyone. If this operation and its aftermath is going to be difficult—and I expect that it will—then I don't want Laura to see me frightened and in pain. I admire Laura's strength, her ability to juggle her schedule so she can work at a difficult job, have time for her children, and still be with me. But I don't want her to see me being weak. Already our relationship has been through enough crises—over her divorce and our desire to live together—during which I have acted foolishly. This time I want to prove that I can be strong, or at least prove that

I can be strong in front of her. On the other hand I am really frightened. Part of me feels that being macho is stupid, that I want her to be there to comfort me.

I resolve the conflict by acting dogmatically independent. Twice already I have told her it isn't necessary for her to be with me. Again in the waiting room she offers to call the office and delay her appointment. I say no in an angry tone.

Simpson comes out into the waiting room to say he'll be with me shortly. As soon as he leaves Laura quips, "You certainly know how to pick handsome doctors." That makes me feel angry and jealous. Leaving, Laura says, "I'm sure it will be a brief meeting. I'll try to be done quickly. If, for some reason I'm late, then wait for me here until I get back."

IN THE LOCKER ROOM, the attendant gives me an ugly green hospital gown and a pair of disposable slippers. She seems frightened of patients. I cannot be certain whether it is her fear or mine I sense. But this, my first experience with the people who do the hospital's routine work, is unsettling.

This morning, as the attendant is locking my clothes away, she wants me to put away my copy of *The New Yorker*. Afraid of waiting on that wooden bench partly naked without anything to read, I start arguing with her. She pulls the magazine out of my hand and puts it in my locker. Sulking, I vow to write an angry letter to the hospital administrator.

I WAS SOON TO FIND that attendants, orderlies, and staff nurses, unlike my physicians, often treated me as just another patient to be dealt with before the day ended. It took me some time to realize it was unreasonable for me to expect reassurance from employees who were frequently earning little more than minimum wage and who were often overworked. By doing unpleasant tasks I'd never consider doing, they created an ordered, hygienic environment in which my doctors had the time to relate to me. Yet, because the staff imposed a routine, I was at first unthinkingly quarrelsome.

SIMPSON IS WEARING an operating costume with folds of cloth around his shoes. It makes him look like an astronaut. From the time I enter the room, Simpson and his two assistants begin a continual risqué patter, which distracts me from my nervousness. I get onto the table in the well-lit antiseptic room. There I am, the center of attention. I've always craved attention, and nothing is as attention-absorbing as lying on an operating table with the lights, doctors, and nurses focused on you. Briefly I feel a rush of pleasure, which vanishes when Simpson tells me to relax. I am jumpy. The table, the instruments, the nurses' hands all feel cold. The whole world seems cold and much too white. I decide to redesign operating rooms so that they have bright colors. Fuck white.

I ask, "When is it going to hurt?"

Simpson takes out a large needle (or maybe it just seems large). "Relax; I'll tell you when it's going to hurt."

I say, "Wait a minute."

"Okay, I'll wait. Tell me when you're ready."

"Okay. I'm ready."

Simpson says, "This is going to hurt. Then, it's going to sting. Then it's going to go numb."

Gail, one of Simpson's two assistants, has large beautiful green eyes. She holds my hand before the pain begins. First it hurts. Then it stings. Then it goes numb. I try to twist around to see when Simpson begins operating, but Gail holds me down. Holding me down is a good idea. Simpson has already opened me up without my realizing it.

Between requesting clamps and assorted surgical tools, Simpson asks about being a journalist. He asks how I get article assignments, why I became interested in agriculture, what I think of the Russian grain deal, what I think of Secretary of Agriculture Earl Butz. Simpson says that he has a friend who is an unemployed writer. "Can you talk to him? Maybe you can help him out, give him some tips?" The operating table is no place to say no. I say that I'd be delighted to talk to him. "Just give him my phone number."

Simpson says, "Tell me when it begins to hurt again. I'm going deeper." I feel the scalpel go past the numb area of my arm and I tell him. He shoots more local anesthetic into my arm. I scream. I didn't know pain could go that deep. Quickly, it gets numb. Interested, I ask detailed questions about the anesthetic, which has the same characteristics and chemical qualities as Novocain. His hand is inside my arm, not hurting but pulling and feeling crowded. He is trying to get a firm grip on the lump so he can cut it out and not leave any inside my arm. I am impatient for him to get it over with. "Did you get it yet? Did you get it yet?" I keep pestering him.

My lump is no longer a lump, a hunk of fatty tissue. It is a tumor. Now I can ask Simpson whether the tumor is benign or malignant. He says that he doesn't know, that Aaron will tell me after it comes back from the lab. Gail asks how long I waited before getting it removed. I tell her and she says, "You shouldn't have waited so long." That frightens me. While sewing me up, Simpson explains that the tumor is a grossly enlarged lymph node.

THE LYMPH NODES (or glands) are part of a system that purifies the blood. One of many such glands located under my right arm became dramatically enlarged, making it a golf-ball-sized tumor. Normally the gland is the size of a fingernail on the smallest finger.

The next step is to send the tumor to a laboratory where a pathologist will look at slides of it to determine its origin. Most tumors removed in a routine biopsy are benign. Benign tumors are harmless and their cause is generally unknown. A malignant tumor reveals under the microscope that it is composed of cancerous cells.

SIMPSON GIVES ME instructions for care of my arm. He says that I can go back to work if I want, that in fact many of his patients return to work immediately after the operation. He says he'll give me a prescription for pain medication, but some patients find that all they need is aspirin.

The operation has taken probably less than half an hour. I am eager to get out of the operating room and out of the building. I dress as quickly as possible, check the waiting room for Laura, and go outside. Outside feels like it has been newly created. I never want to be inside again.

Irrationally, I am angry at Laura for not being there. I sent her away, but now I want her here, immediately. My arm is beginning to hurt and I want the prescription filled and the pain medicine inside me—instantly. I want to go home.

Less than five minutes later, Laura comes rushing down the street. "I'm all right. I'm all right," I say irritably, trying to be firmly in control, answering her questions about the operation in monosyllables. We go to a pharmacy across the street and I want to kill the druggist for taking so long.

Aaron asked me to request slides from Simpson. In addition to sending the tumor to the laboratory for a formal report,

23

Aaron wants personally to look under his microscope at the sample slides, which Simpson has pressed against the tumor. Although I worry about losing lymph nodes, the fear is unwarranted. The body has plenty to spare.

Laura wants to drive me to Aaron's office. "You look weak and shaken up," she says. "It is stupid for you to walk it." I insist, trying to prove that I am in control. Laura realizes it is senseless to argue, so we both walk.

The short three blocks are very long indeed. I introduce Laura to Aaron and hand him the package that Simpson prepared for me. Then I kiss Laura good-bye and flag down a cab, forgetting for a painful instant not to use my right arm. I just want to go home. I want to be alone.

The pain gets worse. At my apartment I turn on the telephone answering machine, trying to cut myself off from the world. I am afraid to look at my wound and delay the unpleasant task of changing the bandage. For the first time in my life, I am disgusted by my own body.

THANKS TO ANESTHETICS, operations don't hurt when they're happening, they hurt after the anesthetic wears off and there is no one around. This is a hard weekend. I have never felt pain before, not for longer than a bruise in a baseball game or the duration of a dentist's drill. Simpson has said that some patients tolerate pain easily and are able to return to work at once. I think of those stoic patients with embarrassment. Clearly most people are stronger and braver than I.

This has been my first entry into the world of surgery, and the massive bandage under my right arm makes clear the reality of the tumor. Before the operation, the tumor was merely a lump, something to be attended to when I got the chance. I refused to think about the seriousness of its consequences. Nothing major could be wrong with me—certainly nothing like cancer. I am twenty-eight years old. I am in good health. I ride my bicycle to get around town, often going miles at a stretch.

I've always felt safe from life's dangers. Like many of my generation, I managed to avoid the war in Vietnam. The most painful event in my life up to now has been the time my wife left me, and that not because I loved her or because the marriage was any good, but because my pride was hurt that *she* was walking out on *me*. I've always seen myself as somehow special, someone whom luck or fate has picked for momentous achievements. Should I have trouble making money, finishing my book on agriculture, or settling down to a life with Laura, I trust that something will come along in time to help me out of the particular difficulty I am in. The idea that I may be faced with a situation that I cannot control and that can change my life seems alien to me.

For me, the pain works as a trigger for emotions I've been unwilling to acknowledge. That weekend I realize for the first time what has been obvious for more than a week: I am waiting for a doctor to tell me whether I have cancer. Suddenly waiting seems intolerable. The more I think about it, the more convinced I become that I am going to die. I hate God, fate, myself, my apartment, my life, and everything else that comes to mind. I am angry.

It has become trite to say that we take out our anger on the ones we love. From my way of looking at things, through the filter of my self-pity, I decide to do Laura a favor: I will break off my relationship with her, sparing her the difficulty of being with a sick and dying man. I will face my grim future alone, quickly finishing my long-overdue book. I invent a role for myself, not realizing it is one that my personality will never be able to sustain. I am going to be quietly brave and die alone, without complaint. The decision made, I feel ebullient as I call Laura and tell her that I never want to see her again. It is a short, quick conversation. She calls back almost immediately asking, "Are you sure?" No, I'm not sure. I feel humiliated. I apologize. Maybe after telling her I don't want her around, this is my dumb way of saying I am lonely, of testing her to see whether she'll really call me back.

"OF COURSE, I knew what you were doing," she told me later. "You were afraid you had cancer and that's how you tried to deal with it. But, even though I knew you didn't really mean it, I was hurt anyway. No, I couldn't just look at what you were doing objectively and say, 'There he goes again.' I was in love with you and you were hurting me."

As it turned out, that call to Laura was the first of a series of impulsive, fear-driven responses to the cancer experience. From time to time, I would find my behavior taken over by some fear or anger that I didn't know was inside me and that I didn't recognize until later, when the lashing out or the self-destruction was over.

ON SUNDAY, May 1, I begin to feel better again. I remove the enormous bandage and notice that the wound is quite small. Inside the wound, Simpson has left an absorbent "wick." He told me to remove it by gently pulling at its string, which I do. Then I put on a fresh gauze bandage and tape. My arm no longer feels confined or quite as stiff. The pain is mostly gone. I am surprised at how minor the operation really was and that I made such a fuss about it.

By Tuesday I am sitting in Aaron's office listening to the diagnosis. He tells me how lucky I am. He says that the tumor was caused by an innocuous disease called toxoplasmosis, which comes from eating steak tartare or playing with cats. It may make me feel a little weak, but it will go away by itself.

"I can't tell you how relieved I am," Aaron says.

"Why, what did you think was wrong with me?"

"Why go into that? You're lucky. You should be grateful that it wasn't serious. That should be enough for you." Aaron's lab assistant takes more blood for a test that will confirm the diagnosis. "I don't think I need to see you again," he says, "but why don't you call the office at the end of the week?"

3

A CONDITION OF RELIVING the past is that one knows what happens next. The relief of being told that I didn't have cancer was unremarkable except for the cancer diagnosis that followed. When Aaron told me the good news, I felt confused. I had been prepared for the worst. For more than a year, Laura had been recommending that I read *On Death and Dying*. Her brother Matthew had taught it in a psychology course. Laura had even met its author, Elisabeth Kübler-Ross and been strongly impressed. I had picked the weekend I was recovering from surgery to finally read the book, deciding that fear was a good incentive for seriously considering—for the first time—the actual possibility that I might die. The fear had made me impulsively willing to leap at pessimism before the news was in, and to attempt to control and prepare myself for some sad and painful future.

Certainly I felt relieved when Aaron told me that I didn't

have cancer. Yet, in a curious way, I felt disappointed, as if the intensity of my feelings was somehow trivialized. Today, I can look back and say that I sensed that Aaron was wrong. And I did. But I'm sure others who have undergone a biopsy have felt a similar sense of foreboding—one that doesn't evaporate instantly when the doctor says you're all right. Good news, like bad, takes a while to sink in. It was only later, when the news changed and I felt caught off guard, that I was angry. When I was ready for the worst, my doctor told me there was nothing to worry about. After I believed him, he told me he had made a mistake.

ON THURSDAY, May 6, 1976, I am at the massive South Building of the U.S. Department of Agriculture researching an article for *The Washingtonian* magazine. A specialist in personnel procedures is explaining to me the hiring policy for the agriculture department, which has more staff protecting forests than serving farmers. We are interrupted by a call from the press secretary informing me that my request for an exclusive interview with Earl Butz has been granted for three-thirty that afternoon.

It is one of the most exciting developments of my professional life. For the past three years, I have been writing about Secretary Butz, reporting on his activities for a newsletter on migrant workers and later for the readers of *The New Republic.* The book I am writing concerns how Butz's decisions have transformed the way America produces food for this country and the world.

Agriculture was a subject I knew nothing about when I began. But the importance of Butz's decisions, within the context of a world food shortage, created a modest demand for journalists who could explain what was happening. To use Butz's pejorative description, I was "an instant expert." Like other reporters new to the field, I began with contempt for Butz, believing that he was corrupt, bigoted, and stupid. My first articles reflected that contempt, so it is a surprise now that he consents to see me—a surprise and, professionally, a gift. He does not know that I have come to have grudging respect for his intelligence and political craftiness. I am excited by the prospect of confronting Butz with the unanswered questions I have been saving for just such an opportunity.

I spend some time in the department's press room, where wire and financial reporters who have been covering agriculture for years give me tips on how to handle Butz. They fill me in on the latest rumors of Butz's losing fight with Henry Kissinger for President Ford's favor and the power to make international food policy. Although I am not used to working with a tape recorder, I decide that this occasion is special. No one in the press room has a loaner. So, having cut the time really fine, I dash home to get the one that I own but that I'm not sure works.

At home, I play back the messages on the telephone answering machine. There are several—all from Aaron Falk's office requesting with increased urgency that I call as soon as I get in. The most recent message is from the doctor himself. I return the call and Aaron comes on almost immediately. "I have to talk to you," he says. "Can you come in right away?"

"No."

"Why not?"

"I have an interview with Earl Butz at three-thirty, and he's more important than you are. Why? What is it?"

"I can't tell you over the phone."

I think, *This can't be happening to me. It's too bizarre. What can't he tell me over the phone? That I have cancer? That I am going to die?* I say, "Why can't you tell me over the phone?"

"I can't. I just can't. Can't you cancel your interview?"

Then I do have cancer. I am going to die. I cannot imagine calling the secretary of agriculture's secretary to say, "I'm sorry, but I have to cancel my three-thirty interview today with Secretary Butz. My doctor wants to tell me in person that I have cancer."

I tell Aaron angrily, "No, I can't cancel the interview. He's the secretary of agriculture."

"Then call me as soon as you're done. I don't care how late it is. I'll be here in my office waiting for your call."

I go to the interview with Butz, hating him because he will live and I won't. I interview him mechanically; it's something I'm able to do because I wrote the questions out in advance and I don't have to think about them—questions about Richard Nixon's plans to abolish the agriculture department, about Butz's plans to move food stamps to the Department of Health, Education and Welfare, about rumors of the secretary's private displeasure with the Soviet oil and grain agreement, about USDA's inability to police the futures markets, about the secretary's tardy knowledge of the grain inspection scandal. I feel as if I am an observer, watching myself ask questions and react to answers with timely follow-ups. Part of me is considering the possibility of my own death, amazed that I can continue with this mundane conversation. Part of me is engaged as a reporter, finally getting to talk to a primary source. But the pleasure of the interview has been lost. It is replaced by the need to cope, to get through the hour until I talk to Aaron. There is no time to adjust to the news that I have cancer, to feel sad and reorient myself to this new reality. First I have to be unemotional to get through this interview. Then I have to see Aaron and get the information.

I AM LIGHTHEADED when I walk into Aaron's office, tape recorder in hand. I feel dazed, as if I've just come from a boxing match. I'm also relieved that I'm away from Earl Butz and the need to mask my emotions. And finally, I'm frightened of what Aaron is going to tell me. I say, "It's cancer isn't it?"

He points to the tape recorder. "Is that thing turned on?"

"No."

"No," he says, "it's not cancer. It's Hodgkin's disease."

FOR WEEKS AFTERWARD Aaron refused to admit that Hodgkin's disease is cancer, saying rather that it's "a disease of the lymphatic system." It was like saying that leukemia isn't cancer but a disease of the blood, or that lung cancer isn't cancer but rather a lung disorder. When I confronted him, he explained, "Most people think that cancer is bound to be fatal and are not sophisticated about the latest techniques. So if I say it's Hodgkin's disease instead of cancer, then frequently the patient hasn't heard of it. In any event, if I don't call it cancer the patient won't automatically assume that it's fatal."

THAT AFTERNOON I say, "I've heard of Hodgkin's disease." I had just read in Kübler-Ross's book the description of a woman who dies from it.

"What have you heard about it?"

I tell him.

He says, "Well, it used to be fatal. Nowadays, tremendous progress has been made in its treatment."

I try to push Aaron into answering questions about my life expectancy. First, however, he wants to explain to me the change in diagnosis between Tuesday and today.

He is shaken. He is embarrassed that he made an error. But there's more to his behavior. In some way that I cannot pinpoint—by his intonation, choice of language, way of looking at me—he is expressing concern for me. He is sad that he has to give me this news. He knows that whatever my future, what he's told me is difficult for anyone to hear.

RECENTLY, AARON said, "Patients have different ways of adjusting to their disease. Illness threatens people. A new uncontrollable mysterious force enters their lives, and trying to control that force, I think, is an automatic reaction. It is like standing at the bottom of a hill and all of a sudden there's an avalanche. You put up your hands to stop it, to halt the flow of the rocks."

AARON EXPLAINS that over the weekend he looked at the "touch-preps"—the slides Simpson had pressed against the tumor—and didn't like what he saw. So he was relieved when the pathologist said that it was toxoplasmosis. "I'm sorry," he says. "I should have waited to check out all my hunches before giving you that diagnosis on Tuesday." The blood test was negative, demonstrating that the toxoplasmosis diagnosis was incorrect. Aaron returned to the pathologists at George Washington University Hospital.

HODGKIN'S DISEASE requires skill to diagnose. A pathologist has to be familiar with the disease, which—when the cancerous tumor is sliced and put under the microscope—shows the distinctive "Sternberg-Reed cell," a giant organism containing two huge nuclei. Aaron later explained, "It's very simple. Either you have a Sternberg-Reed cell or you don't. In your case the pathologist did not see the Sternberg-Reed cell at first, because cutting a tumor is like cutting a slice of salami. The first slice he took didn't have it, so he took another slice, and he took finer slices."

AARON PROCEEDS with the story of what happened: "I told the pathology department at G. W., 'This is a very serious matter. Before I tell Mr. Solkoff I want to make sure that each of you looks at his slides and that you unanimously confirm the diagnosis and will put it in writing.' " He hands me the report. "Examination of thinner sections reveals Hodgkin's disease." He says that he wanted other opinions, so he went across town and to Bethesda, Maryland, to show my slides to pathologists at Georgetown University Hospital and at the National Institutes of Health. He hands me another report. "I wanted to make sure that the diagnosis was confirmed by some of the best pathologists in the country. I wanted to be absolutely certain when I told you that I have no doubt in my mind that you have Hodgkin's disease."

As a reporter, I appreciate his impressive legwork. He was diligent and thorough. I also realize that I'm lucky. If Aaron hadn't insisted on checking and double-checking, then perhaps I would have had to wait for another tumor and another biopsy until a pathologist finally identified the disease. By then the cancer could have spread even farther. I realize that Aaron may have saved my life. I realize that instead of being pleased by his efforts, Aaron is still embarrassed by the original error, which was not even his. However, I am too impatient to spend time reassuring Aaron. I ask, "Will it kill me?"

He squirms.

I ask, "What are my chances of surviving this disease?"

That he can answer. "I don't know."

$$\boxed{4}$$

ACCORDING TO the American Cancer Society, with the filing of Tissue Examination Number S76-1606 I became one of the 675,000 Americans who were diagnosed as having cancer in 1976. That year Hodgkin's disease killed 3,200 Americans. Although it is relatively rare, this cancer attracts considerable attention because so many of its victims are children and young adults and because, historically, medical and popular literature has focused on its being inevitably fatal. Although odds for survival and even cure have changed dramatically in recent years, its grim reputation persists. Also, patients still die from it. In 1976 doctors certified that Hodgkin's disease was the cause of death for 193 men and women in the 25–29-year age category—my category.

THAT AFTERNOON, Thursday, May 6, 1976, there is much to decide.

Aaron suggests that I might want a second opinion. He offers to give me the slides and the pathologists' reports so I can take the information to another physician. I know the advantage of second opinions. When I had a back problem in college, one of the physicians at Columbia's clinic recommended an operation. I consulted another doctor—a specialist in back disorders—and was told that an operation was unnecessary. I followed the specialist's advice, and the problems the first doctor suggested never developed.

However, this situation is different. Aaron didn't make the diagnosis; a pathologist did. And Aaron has already solved the problem of getting additional opinions by going to several pathologists. I ask Aaron, "What will happen if I get a second opinion?"

He explains that there are many fine physicians in Washington, that if I consult one the doctor will take my slides, give them to a pathologist, and after receiving the pathologist's report he will proceed to the next step.

I say, "Do you think enough pathologists have looked at my slides?"

"Yes."

"Is there any chance that another pathologist will say that it isn't Hodgkin's disease."

"No."

"I gather from the number of pathologists you've seen that the odds are high that even if I get a second opinion, the second doctor is likely to show my slides to a pathologist who's already seen them."

"I'd say that is highly likely."

"Then what's the advantage of getting a second opinion? It seems to me that I'd just be wasting time."

"I don't think there's any advantage. But generally it's a

good idea to get a second opinion, and I think I should offer you that option."

"I don't think it's necessary. What do I do now?"

Aaron explains that before he treats the disease, it is first necessary to know where it is located—a process called "staging." Although only one tumor was discovered, it is possible that the disease has spread throughout my body. Since the lymphatic system is circulatory, it is necessary to do tests along different parts of the system. The good news is that I currently do not have any of the apparent disease symptoms, such as night sweats, itching, loss of weight, or pain when I drink alcohol. The chest X rays show no tumors. My blood is all right. However, Aaron does need to do additional tests to see whether my bone marrow, spleen, and liver are cancerous (the word he uses is "negative"). When he has the results, then he can prescribe a form of treatment and tell me about my life chances. He describes the tests. First a bone-marrow biopsy will be done in his office. Then Simpson will perform exploratory surgery, removing my spleen and samples of my liver. That will require a week to ten days of hospitalization. Removal of the spleen, he says, is a routine procedure. Like the appendix, it is not a vital organ. "Plenty of people live long lives without a spleen."

"Like rodeo cowboys," I say, remembering my reporting on a rodeo and meeting a cowboy in Oklahoma City whose spleen had been removed after a bucking bronco had stepped on him.

Aaron says, "We have to do all of this quickly, so we can begin treatment as soon as possible."

AARON REALIZED the importance of maintaining my morale. He feared that when I left his office I was going to be flooded by pessimistic information about Hodgkin's disease—information that, while incorrect, might depress me and discourage my undergoing necessary treatment.

My 1975 encyclopedia, for example, says of Hodgkin's disease, "Complete recovery is extremely rare." The District of Columbia public library's medical and science reference books, which five years later are still on the shelf, are consistently gloomy. One text notes: "The disease is invariably fatal, usually within five years of the onset. . . ." Dick Francis, one of my favorite mystery writers, used my disease in his 1972 thriller *Smokescreen*. "When you went out to look at those two young chasers in her paddock," a character explains, "Nerissa told me what is the matter with her. . . . Some ghastly thing called Hodgkin's disease, which makes her glands swell, or something, and turn cellular, whatever that really means. She doesn't know very clearly herself, I don't think. Except that it is absolutely fatal."

Even some physicians still refuse to believe that a patient can survive Hodgkin's disease. In the 1980 edition of his standard medical textbook on the subject, Dr. Henry Kaplan sadly admits, "The concept of Hodgkin's disease as inevitably fatal has continued to be handed down in medical teaching, almost to the present day, with the consequence that many physicians still hold so firmly to this conviction that they react emotionally to any suggestion that it is no longer true."

That afternoon, Aaron counseled me against reading about the disease because popular medical literature and basic textbooks have not kept up with the advances. When I pressured him, saying that I have difficulty believing something unless it is in print, he suggested that I call the American Cancer Society for a recent brochure and promised to lend me journal articles. (The journal articles, I found, were incomprehensible—discussions on "MOPP versus the 3 and 2 technique for total nodal irradiation.")

In retrospect, that Thursday afternoon meeting with Aaron was more important than I realized. Even though he refused to use the word, cancer terminology crept into his explanations, and we both knew that cancer was what I had. More significant than telling me I had cancer, though, was whether I would trust other people to use their professional skills to try to save my life. It was Aaron's intention that afternoon to foster in me the hope that the medical establishment could treat my disease. Less important than whether he or another physician treated me was whether I was going to allow myself to be treated. I cannot imagine a more difficult situation—for a doctor or for anyone else—than to convince someone to take the action necessary to save his or her life.

At that time I was not one who normally trusted specialists or established procedures. However, I had a cancer that frequently can be checked or even cured by conventional forms of treatment—radiation and chemotherapy. It is a cancer where initial treatment can be vital. If, for some reason, my dose levels weren't high enough, or if the treatment were not successful the first time around, then my chances of survival would drop dramatically. That afternoon Aaron convinced me to trust in the medical establishment and in competent specialists. And he convinced me without my realizing that I'd been convinced of anything. The fact that I knew Aaron for only thirteen days made the extent of my trust all the more remarkable.

5

DIRECTLY ACROSS the street from Aaron's office is a large apartment building with a very dark and empty bar. I am sitting there alone, aware that the place satisfies some internal stereotype. Stirring the ice cubes in my Scotch, I am unprepared for this moment. I'm barely sipping the Scotch. An event of this magnitude deserves serious drinking, but I don't want to get drunk.

I feel obliged to be alone, aware that from now on my world is going to be different. I force myself to think about my cancer and my feelings about it. Before I tell anyone else or see anyone else, I want to get a better sense of my own reactions. My instinct is to run to Laura and hold her—not to talk but just to be held. I am restless and confined. I want to walk for miles, to escape myself. Smoking a cigarette that is burning too slowly, I try to impose a sense of discipline upon myself.

I consider the information Aaron has just given me. I

have a disease of the lymphatic system, and I don't really know what the lymphatic system is. My doctor won't know whether the disease will kill me until he does some tests. The tests will be painful, and that frightens me.

I am disturbed by the uncertainty. If Aaron can tell me with any assurance either that I will definitely die in two years or that I will definitely live, it will be easier to deal with. Not knowing whether I will live or die seems even worse than the idea of dying. I am not in the mood for an existential crisis. Like most adolescents, I went through one in high school (when Kierkegaard was in fashion). I'd prefer delaying the next one until I am sixty-five or seventy. I am too busy trying to get some stability in my career and my relationship with Laura to concern myself with the meaning of life. This cancer is imposing some sort of spiritual test, a test I don't want to take, a test I fear I've already failed.

I feel cheated. Aaron cheated me out of an appropriate reaction by telling me on Thursday what he should have told me on Tuesday. More to the point, I feel cheated of the right to lead a normal healthy life.

I do not feel like praying. Some get comfort, unity, or guidance in prayer. But I have trouble getting beyond the words, and so prayer feels uncomfortable.

My religious education has been literal and strict. The God of my people reduces one's lifespan in half if one doesn't observe the rituals of Passover. He does equally unmerciful things if one breaks the commandments (especially the one on honoring one's parents), as my mother has reminded me with some frequency during our angry phone calls. I believe in God but not that God. I believe in a God who is merciful and loving, who wants the world to be run with compassion, justice, and peace. I believe that God wants us to be His instruments for good, and that He is altogether too sensible to interfere with the lives of individuals. I find it hard to imagine God counting up sins, answering prayers, or failing to rely on people's God-given skills to solve their own problems. On the other hand, whatever primitive parts of us fear the darkness and the unknown seem to be working inside me on that spring afternoon. I feel myself a helpless victim of God's wrath. Feeling that not only frightens me, it makes me angry. How dare God treat me this way?

Sometimes being alone can make you very self-conscious, as if the whole world were watching in judgment. Popular imagery comes to mind: John Wayne crossing the Red River, James Bond shooting it out with SMERSH, Humphrey Bogart outwitting the Nazis. I am frustrated by a sense of occasion, that my reaction to this Significant Event must live up to certain standards of how a man is supposed to react when faced with danger and death. What I am experiencing is not melodrama, yet the task of facing myself does not lend itself to quiet contemplation. I want to prove something to myself, to behave according to some acceptable standard, and all that comes to mind is melodrama. I make lists of things I enjoy and want to do before I die—more Mozart, more Bach, more Yeats, a trip in a hot-air balloon. I regret not having more fun, not making love to Laura more frequently, not racing fast cars, sailing in regattas, climbing mountains, not seeing sunsets from tropical beaches. Why did I never learn how to play the piano or speak French or play poker? Regret for lost poker games seems somehow undignified.

My humor has always had a black tinge to it. I am amused that I regard this event as a test of my manhood and that I envision my fight with cancer as a movie scene with Errol Flynn fighting the pirates. I resolve to treat my disease as something that is not especially serious, which I will dismiss with flip, self-deprecating comments. My emotions are on a roller coaster. I am suddenly afraid that I will remain trapped in my aloneness and in my disappointment over who I am and what I feel. I want to be reassured that there is someone out there, that I am loved. Frantically, I call Laura. She hasn't left work yet. We meet, but instead of holding her and weeping, which is what I want to do, I become cold and logical. "This is what he said," I say. "This is what is going to happen," I say. We both know that control has failed to hide my fear.

FOR SOME REASON, I assumed that fear of death was going to be my problem. I heard what Aaron said, I weighed the evidence, and I figured I was going to survive. I assumed there would be grim moments, that the experience ahead was going to be awful. I realized that death was a possibility; I considered death. But death seemed too unreal, something that happened to others. I was not going to die. I knew that, finally and absolutely. It was a knowledge that I am still unsure about: was I being prophetic or self-deluded?

I was certainly not prepared for other people thinking that I was going to die, not Laura, nor my parents, nor many of my friends. Suddenly, those closest to me changed their behavior toward me. Preoccupied with myself, I often refused to see or understand why their behavior changed.

I have since learned that the experience of having cancer cannot be explained. In *The Looking Glass War*, John le Carré's spy says to himself, "Nothing ever bridged the gulf between the man who went and the man who stayed behind." No one I knew had been where I was—not my doctors, my friends, my relatives. My fight with cancer turned out to be an adventure, like participating in a war or exploring virgin territory. It was not until later that I realized the extent of my loneliness and alienation.

6

FOLLOWING AARON'S SUGGESTION, on Friday, May 7, I look up the number in the D.C. phone book and dial.

"Good morning, American Cancer Society. May I help you?"

"Yes, I'd like some information on cancer, specifically Hodgkin's disease."

The society has a pamphlet listing how many people get cancer each year and another describing Hodgkin's disease. "Will that do?"

She takes down my name and address. Then she asks, "Why do you want this information?"

"Because I was just diagnosed as having Hodgkin's disease."

There is a long pause. Then she starts speaking too quickly, repeating my name and address and the titles of publications she will send "right away." Nervously, she says, "Is there anything else I can do for you?"

"I don't know. Are there any services the American Cancer Society provides for cancer patients I should know about?"

"Just the pamphlets," she blurts, saying a fast "goodbye," hanging up the phone before I have time to respond. [Years later, I'd find out about a program where Cancer Society volunteers drive cancer patients to and from treatment. Knowledge of that, as I'd discover, would have been a godsend.]

The phone call gives me an uneasy feeling: the people working for the American Cancer Society are afraid of cancer patients. Do they know something I don't know? I shrug off the incident, determined to believe that friends and family will take the news more rationally.

I was wrong.

FIVE YEARS is a long time. Yet remembering that phone call five years ago just plunged me into a sadness. It is like being in some alien world—a mirror image of this one, except that I feel isolated, surrounded by a thick foglike substance interfering with my ability to touch people or even objects. Flies buzz around the typewriter. The air-conditioner growls. The digits on the clock change as I watch: 10:33, 10:34, 10:35. . . . I am unable to understand the meaning of time or to remove myself from this position of watching and waiting, alone—forever trapped.

At some level of consciousness I realize that I am healthy now. I am cured.

Emotionally, this act of remembrance is a return to despair, to an overwhelming sensation that my true self has been stripped of all pretense, that I know who I really am and that the real me is hollow, valueless.

The despair disappears when I go to lunch, talk to Diana about our wedding plans, write about agriculture, utility investments, the Trust Indenture Act, or anything that is not cancer and how I've survived it.

Survival is a curious word. I have survived the disease. There is a small scar under my right arm and a large one down the center of my abdomen. Two one-inch scars are faded on the tops of my feet. A small blue pinpoint—a tattoo made as a target for radiation therapy—remains at the base of my chest. Otherwise, I am unmarked by the effects of the disease or its treatment. You could not tell by looking or by my level of activity that I once had cancer.

Concentration on 1976 causes me to grieve over my love for Laura, over the realization, slow in coming, that the despair the cancer brought killed our relationship.

I believed I would live. She believed I would die. She hid her belief. Facts could not shake her belief, nor alter her despair. I had my own despair, my own hopelessness to deal with. I was unable to see hers. We reached across the gulf of our misperceptions, hoping to hide our true feelings. But the sadness steadily blocked our ability to bridge the gulf. We gave each other comfort and love. But I couldn't give her hope. She couldn't give me honesty. After a while, the comforts we gave could not compensate for our deficiencies. The pain we caused each other—but which mostly I caused her— was intensified by sickness's daily burden of insensitivity and self-centeredness. Eventually, the pain was too great to forgive, and forgetting became impossible.

Laura once said to me, "You didn't like having cancer, but you liked it in a way. I think you liked to use it as a way of shocking people, like me. You could manipulate me a lot with it.

"You were scared. You were real scared. I figured if I was scared, you were *really* scared. I was terrified, because it's frightening. Cancer is frightening. It's frightening when it's someone you care about. I was also angry. There were lots of reasons why I was angry. One reason was because I figured that there was going to be a lot of responsibility put on me. I mean it wasn't that clearly thought out at the time, but I felt that, and I was angry. And I was angry that this thing was happening to you.

"My way of dealing with things," she said, "is to take care of people. I knew that was a lot of what I'd be doing. I can't say that it comes naturally to me, but I feel like I have to take care of people because of some whatever-it-was in my upbringing."

ONE EXCITING DAY in the spring of 1976, a white shag rug arrives at Laura's house from Sloan's. Her kids call Laura at work. Luke, at ten, is pretending masculine indifference. Timothy, eight, and Karen, seven, are unabashedly enthusiastic, grabbing the phone from each other, talking a mile a minute, describing the rug as well as the ornate sofa for three (with a peacock spreading its wings in the textile) and the mirrored coffee table, which Laura will religiously shine thrice daily with bargain-brand window cleaner from Safeway.

The white rug forms an island in the big rambling house in Chevy Chase, where the roof leaks and the dust of months of neglected housekeeping remains undisturbed in little piles. The island represents Laura's dream that she can put her life in order. She uses the word *struggle* to describe her attempt. Sometimes she lets me know that I, too, am part of her dream, sitting next to her on the peacock sofa.

Laura's anger is part of her "struggle" and her personality. She is especially angry at the house, she says, because it is a symbol of everything else she's angry about—her life, her marriage, the number of her children, men, the Roman Catholic Church, her family, not going to law school. Sometimes I am uncertain whether her language indicates anger or is a conscious self-parody of her anger, at which we both can laugh. Punchy, often dated mixtures of obscenities, curses, and curious expressions stream out of her. "Motherfucker" is a favorite. Its meaning changes with intonation. A motherfucker is someone she likes, hates, who does something she disapproves of. She says things like "Stick it in your ear," "Not on your tintype," "What's it to you, Ollie?"

EARLY in our relationship, I gave her a ticket so we could meet for a weekend together in New Orleans after my research into rice farming in Arkansas and Louisiana. Drinking too many rum "hurricanes," I react to the combination of her earthy language, anger, and fury during our lovemaking, which had the intensity of seized pleasure. "Sometimes you frighten me," I said.

She grabbed her blue jeans from the floor, jumped straight up in the center of the enormous hotel bed, and began hitching up her pants. "I'm sick of men being afraid of me. You idiot, my anger is progress. For years I was angry and didn't realize it. Now I can express my anger, how totally pissed off I am by all those years I was screwed by life and by my fucking husband and by everyone and everything. Finally I get the courage to open my mouth after years of being a good daughter and a good wife and a good mother. Finally I can say that I'm angry at getting screwed and I'm not going to let anyone fuck me over anymore, but you fucking men are intimidated by a woman who's honest and says what she means.

"Well, I'm the most exciting woman you'll ever meet," she said, walking off the bed and reaching for her blouse. "But if I'm too much woman for you to handle, and if you can't take it, then buzz off. Because I don't want a man who's frightened of me. If you don't have the balls," she said, starting to leave the room at three o'clock in the morning, "to handle an honest woman who's not about to pretend that she isn't angry when she's been fucked over by life, then you can buzz off. Who needs you?"

By rushing to the doorway, blocking her exit, I stopped her from walking out of my life. I calmed her down, which I became good at doing. She was right. She was the most exciting woman I'd ever met. Her anger also frightened me, but that fear I could deal with. At one sober moment near morning, being together became very tender—she cried on my chest as I held her gently. Soon I realized that this tough, aggressive, supercompetent woman, career person, mother, is also very vulnerable. She is, among other things, vulnerable to me.

WE BOTH REALIZE that Laura's relationship with me is an expression of her anger. I am young—seven and one-half years younger than she—and she's convinced that my existence infuriates Jim, her former husband. I'm Jewish, and her mother—who sleeps with a crucifix with a vial of Lourdes water pasted onto the back—does not like Jews. When we met, Laura was still married, and we both feared our relationship would get caught up in the divorce proceedings.

I too am using our relationship. For my parents, Laura's religion, age, and children provoked disapproval. In February, when I told Mother I planned to marry Laura, she said, "I'd prefer you dead." My father said, "If you plan on going ahead with this, I will disown you. On the day of your marriage to this woman, you will no longer be my son." I was using Laura to help me gain independence, especially from Mother. During most of my childhood my mother alone, as a divorced parent, cared for and supported me and arranged for my education. Mother and I had been close—too close. I was a Mamma's boy. After twenty-eight years, my relationship with Laura was helping to distance me from Mother. Finally, I was able to make clear to Mother that my goals for my life are different from hers.

Laura and I both suspect that our love is greater than the utilitarian value of our relationship. We plan to find out. Her divorce decree neutralizes me as a danger. Early in April, Father and I reached an understanding. Phone calls with Mother are becoming increasingly cordial. My parents acknowledge they have no choice but to accept. This summer, when Jim takes the children, Laura and I will live together. We will test whether our love, which flourished under difficulties, can survive tranquillity. We are aware of this seeming paradox. We are, after all, a couple in an age of ubiquitous therapy; we talk to each other about her fears of men and my fears of women and our hopes for a future together.

The cancer diagnosis comes along at a turning point in our relationship. We're not stupid. We know that. And it's frightening. Why now? What will it do to us?

Laura says that the white rug is a symbol of her fighting back. After ten years of "mindlessly submitting," she realized that she hated life with Jim, that three children were enough, that she might not have professional skills but she was going out on the job market, into the "real world" and make a life for herself. "People say I'm crazy for wanting a white rug, that you can't keep it clean. But I've always wanted a white rug, and just because they don't have the balls it takes to maintain it, I'll show them." She does, making the rug and sofa off limits to the cats and to children who don't wash their hands or who try to consume a Twinkie or soda in the area she continally patrols, vacuums, and shines. (Outside that area, Laura's indifference to housework is even greater than mine. That upsets her. Rather than minding, I find it makes me feel more relaxed.)

I admire Laura for her struggle. When we met two years ago at the Migrant Legal Action Program, she was a secretary. Unlike others, she typed quickly and efficiently and avoided the office politics that pervaded the place. When the administrative assistant left, Laura was offered the job. It required that she learn bookkeeping, office management, and the daily details of running a tax-exempt corporation. She was frightened by the necessity of learning a lot quickly and by the sudden responsibility. But her mind is quick. She's ambitious. And the additional money offered more independence. She found it difficult trying something new and conquering fear of failure. I helped, encouraging her, reminding her of her intelligence and ability to handle practical problems.

Then, right before my cancer diagnosis, Laura got a better job. She feels that perhaps she might even fulfill her ambition and go to law school. She bought the furniture from Sloan's, for immediate delivery. Taking her newly acquired credit cards, she arranges a vacation in Puerto Rico for herself and the children. With the excitement of a child who's just seen magic for the first time, she says, "This is the first time I've ever been able to take the kids anywhere."

After telling her about my cancer, she says, "Why don't

you come? I'll pay for it. I haven't used my Carte Blanche card yet. You can get the bone-marrow biopsy next week, when you go into the hospital."

She can't afford it, and anyway I don't want to go. I have work to do. There are seventeen days between diagnosis and the hospital, and I need to prepare myself. I can't spare five days.

The day before the Puerto Rico trip I ask Laura, "Are you going to tell the children?" Without saying anything to her, I hoped that she would keep the news a secret.

"I already have."

"What did they say?"

"Well, you know them. It's hard to get their attention for anything. When they settled down long enough for me to tell them, they said they were sorry and hoped you get well soon."

YEARS LATER, Laura told me that she explained to the children about the lump under my arm, how at first the doctors thought it was nothing, then they discovered it was cancer. She told them I'd have to go into the hospital for an operation and then for treatment. "They all wanted to know whether you were going to die."

"What did you tell them?"

"I told them, 'Yes, he is going to die.' "

LAURA'S CHILDREN have always been a major issue in our relationship. She loves them. From the beginning, she felt guilty that seeing me might endanger custody. She also felt guilty that our relationship was taking time away from them. I admire how Laura gives her children a sense of freedom and joy I never had. Her sense of love means not imposing guilt on them; it is an effort she makes consciously and, in general, successfully. Laura once said, "I was raised to feel guilty. I'm so bored feeling guilty I could scream. That's one thing I'm not going to saddle on my kids."

I know that if Laura and I are ever going to settle down to a life together, I'll have to be a father to the children. Fathering, I know, is difficult enough, but being a father to children who already have one is very difficult indeed. I'll have to be a stepfather who is sensitive to the children's love for their biological father, who lives in the same town and sees them every summer and every other weekend. I know about the difficulties because in my adolescence I had two stepfathers in rapid succession, each unsuited for the job. Since I disliked my own stepfathers, I do not relish becoming one. When I brace myself for the task, I think that maybe, just maybe, I can do it, avoiding the mistakes I've seen firsthand.

From the beginning, dealing with the children was not easy. Because the final decree took so long, the children continued to hope that the divorce would never go through. Luke later told me, "When Mother first started going out with you, it used to make me mad. I mean, I always thought, *Wouldn't it be nice if my mother got back together with my father?* I never really thought it would happen, but I kept a hope that it would. Your being there kind of ruined it."

Tim and Karen rarely agreed with Luke about anything. In opposition to me the three were united. The children, strong-willed and energetic, frequently decided that loyalty to their father required rude behavior.

I realized that I couldn't be both a suitor and a disciplinarian. I couldn't reprimand the children when I was trying to make love to their mother. When the children misbehaved,

I smiled, hoping the smile would be interpreted as an act of neutrality, that I was uninvolved and was not going to be provoked. When they went too far, I'd light a cigarette and frown, letting Laura administer the discipline.

At the beginning of my relationship with Laura, my money situation was pretty good, so I took the family out to plays and expensive dinners. I soon found that going out with all three children at the same time meant disaster. They'd fight among themselves in the car and in the restaurant. Then they'd fight with Laura when she started to break up the fighting.

On one particularly awful outing, I decided to take everyone out in one rowboat along the Chesapeake and Ohio Canal. I insisted on sitting at the stern—the position of navigational power. Although Laura can't swim, I assumed that as long as she had her life jacket on and I was there, she wouldn't worry. The children, however, refused to put on their life jackets. "Daddy never makes us put them on."

"We're not going anywhere unless you put them on," I shouted. The grumbling continued for a while, so I decided to seize the oars, rocking the boat in the process and scaring Laura. Finally the children put on the life jackets. I then returned the oars, and a measure of order was restored. Laura, however, did not like my yelling at the children. She said, "You acted dictatorial." I didn't like Laura's disapproval. When we were alone, we argued about that.

Of the three, I get along best with Luke. Because Luke is interested in politics, we have a lot to talk about. He thinks it "neat" that I am a writer, and he asks detailed questions about reporting. In that hideous battle for the children's loyalty—a battle in which I try to stay scrupulously neutral—Luke generally sides with his mother. I understand Luke's sense of conflict—his love for mother and his guilty feelings toward father. (After all, I felt that way when I was his age.) When he is with his brother and sister, Luke is generally the one to start fights and to be most openly belligerent toward me. But when we are alone, I find it easy to be with him and to do things we both like.

Luke remembered learning about my disease. "First I felt bad and I felt that it was scary and everything. I felt sorry for Mom. I mean, I felt bad for you too. It made me angry that the doctors said it was nothing and you had been real relieved and then they told you you had Hodgkin's disease. I thought it was bad to do that to you. Also Mom was relieved when she found out the lump was nothing. Then when they told you you had Hodgkin's disease and they told you that you were going to die, I knew it was going to be hard on Mom if you died.

"I didn't know what to do to comfort you. I was afraid I'd offend you. You can't really say anything like 'It's okay,' because it's not okay. So I tried to comfort Mom.

"I always thought you were doing to die, that your lymph nodes were all going to get cancerous. Is that what happens when you die of it? I was afraid to ask how you were going to die because I was afraid that it wasn't the right kind of question to ask. Whenever I saw you, I was reminded, *This person's sick and he's going to die.* That scared me.

"It always made me think that I might get cancer. Not that I'd get it from you. It just made me think, *What would happen if I got it?* Just thinking that I was this person who was going to die made me feel real sad. I was trying to think about the way I'd feel, and I'd probably be depressed all the time. Just the thought of those things I wanted to do but couldn't do because I was going to die depressed me—like getting a college degree or becoming a fireman or playing with my friends.

That's when I wanted to be a veterinarian. I thought that if I was going to die, I wouldn't be able to do that."

One of the really bad mistakes I made was not telling Laura's children about my cancer. I should have taken them aside, one by one, and told them what was likely to happen to me and what that meant about my chances for survival. That way I could have dealt with them directly, letting them know that I wasn't afraid of their questions.

Instead, I missed an important opportunity to get close to the children. I made them feel that something mysterious was happening that they shouldn't ask about. One day, I was their mother's boyfriend, who they generally resented and occasionally liked. The next day, I was the object of pity and awe—someone who was going to die. Suddenly, the children didn't know how to act toward me. They were afraid to get angry at me and too scared to be friendly.

I stopped thinking of the children as individuals. I thought of them as "the children." Afraid of how "the children" might react, I became insensitive. I felt that I didn't have the skill, the time, or the energy to deal with them. In effect I said, "These are Laura's children. Let her handle it."

After they were told, they began to look at me as if I were an oddity like a circus freak. The last time I saw them before entering the hospital, I rode my bicycle over to the house. Because they had visited my apartment on Capitol Hill, the children knew how long the ride was. Previously, whenever I bicycled, I'd be bombarded with questions about my trip and about bicycling technique and safety. That evening, there were no questions and the children each announced that they had something to do in their rooms. The next time I saw them was at the hospital after the operation.

7

W E ARE NEARLY contemporaries," Aaron told me after I was cured. "And, yes, I was worried that you might die."

Without treatment, the odds of my being alive by 1981 were 5.8 percent. With treatment, my odds were 40 percent.* My scheduled tests were to categorize the severity of cancer, according to the number of places in my body it was located, using a staging system ranging from I to IV (roman numerals are the traditional style). Staging was not only to tell whether my odds were better or worse than the average range, it was

---

* According to information published in 1972 by the National Cancer Institute (NCI), the average five-year survival rate for all Hodgkin's disease patients *was* 40 percent. That was based on individuals diagnosed from 1960 to 1963. The average survival figures according to stages are from "The Management of Hodgkin's Disease," by Henry S. Kaplan and Saul A. Rosenberg, published in *Cancer* magazine, August, 1975. By 1976, it was already clear that tremendous progress in treatment had been made that was not yet reflected in the

also to determine the most appropriate treatment. If no other cancer was found, I would be a Stage I. My odds of surviving five years would be 86 percent. I'd be given radiation treatment. If Aaron found cancer in my bone marrow or if Simpson found cancer in samples of my liver, then I'd be a Stage IV. My changes of living until 1981 would be 39 percent. I'd be given extensive chemotherapy.

ON WEDNESDAY, May 12, I drive alone to Aaron's office for a bone-marrow biopsy. He is flustered. "You're not scheduled until tomorrow. If you want I can give it to you now. I'm not set up for it, but that won't take long. It makes more sense for you to come tomorrow when I'm ready. Can you come tomorrow?"

"Yes."

"Are you sure you don't mind?"

"Yes."

"Look, it will make more sense if you don't come alone. You may be a little groggy when I'm done. Can you have a friend drive you home?"

"I guess so."

That night Laura calls from Puerto Rico to find out how the test has gone. "Aaron got the date wrong. Tomorrow I'll get pierced."

---

statistics. During that year, the NCI published five-year average survival rates of 54 percent. By 1980, survival increased to 67 percent, representing substantial progress in all stages of the disease. Although Stage IV continues to be serious, Dr. Vincent T. DeVita, director of the NCI, noted, "The major consequence of the development of MOPP chemotherapy for Hodgkin's disease is the demonstration that drugs can cure patients with advanced disease. . . ." MOPP is an acronym for four drugs used in the treatment of cancer.

She says, "The kids are real concerned about you. They keep asking me about you. . . . They're having a great time on the beach, collecting buckets of coconuts and shells. Tim has elaborate plans for painting all this stuff. I may have to lug home half of Puerto Rico." She disregarded warnings about the hot Caribbean sun. Her sunburn was so painful she almost fainted and had to be taken to the hospital. "I was a real asshole," she says. "I love you."

ROBERT, who has been my friend since the first grade, drives me to Aaron's office at 3:45 the following afternoon. Aaron describes the marrow-removal process as "similar to coring an apple." The image is nauseating. Aaron injects Demerol, a synthetic form of morphine, to reduce pain. It causes me to hallucinate slightly. I love the stuff. It separates me from my body. I begin singing: "Row, row, row your boat, gently down the stream . . ." As Aaron turns me around on the examining table, I describe the sensation of floating. "I feel marvelous." Maureen, a resident from George Washington University Hospital, helps Aaron position and hold down my body. "May I hold your hand?" I start flirting, telling her how beautiful she is. "Your skin is so soft and touchable," I say.

Does Aaron disapprove of my outrageous conduct? Is he amused?

He produces a ghastly packet of equipment. The tools look like twelfth-century torture devices. "Don't look," he says. I look anyway and am instantly sorry.

He is holding the largest needle I have ever seen. He is going to put that needle into my right hip. "Don't. I'm not ready. Don't do it."

"Don't look at me. Look forward." Lying on my front, I

am squeezing the hell out of Maureen's hand. Up is the window. I am floating up, through the window, past the bushes and the birds and above the traffic on L Street. But my body—which must belong to someone else—is feeling sharp, turning, unrelenting pain.

Aaron's needle enters the bone in my hip. Turning it, he is removing a piece of marrow. I try to scream, but the scream is stuck in my throat.

"I want to scream," I say.

Aaron says, "Go ahead and scream, but don't turn around."

His permission makes it possible. A scream emerges from my mouth. My body wants to leave the pain on the table and go elsewhere, but Aaron and Maureen are holding it down. My mind floats outside the window on this nice spring day. . . .

"Show me," I say.

Aaron suggests that I might not want to see it.

"Show me anyway."

He is holding my bone marrow with large tweezers. He puts it into a tube. The marrow looks like a diseased worm. I feel sick.

ROBERT WANTS to drop me off at my house and go back to work. My small, slightly seedy one-bedroom apartment is a mess, and I don't want to face it. In the living room, reaching nearly up to the fifteen-foot ceiling, is an enormous stack of *The Washington Post*—papers that after two years I have not yet gotten around to reading, clipping, and filing. The bedroom and living room, separated by a pair of louver doors, looks like one giant mass of papers. Shoved under the bookcases and piled on top of the four-drawer legal-size filing cabinet are press releases from the Department of Agriculture—hog reports, dairy price reports, sugar and sweetener reports, figures on crop yields in the Soviet Union, summaries of international grain prices, surveys on soil erosion in Iowa, population studies on farm workers, pamphlets on raising catfish in Arkansas and on discouraging birds from eating rice crops. The bookshelves need dusting. If I ever get the papers off the floor, vacuuming would be useful. I have let several days go by without doing the dishes, and the kitchen is crawling with roaches. Because I take showers, I haven't scrubbed out the bathtub in months.

Robert's apartment is neat and comfortable. I want to go there. I want to talk. I am still high on Demerol, and I want to describe every detail of the bone-marrow biopsy. Robert drives me to his place and phones work to take the rest of the day off.

I have forgotten how squeamish Robert is until it's too late, after he returns from the bathroom looking slightly green. He later told me, "I was frightened out of my mind. After all, you're my oldest friend. I couldn't face the idea of your being sick and dying. I just didn't want to deal with it."

"IF YOUR BONE MARROW, God forbid, had been positive," Aaron recently told me, "no other studies would have been done. You wouldn't have had a liver-spleen scan. You wouldn't have had a lymphangiogram. You would not have been splenectomized. You wouldn't have had anything. It would have been unnecessary. Because bone marrow involvement would have made you a Four. That observation alone would have dictated a specific therapy. No other diagnostic information would have been helpful."

The good news meant that I had to take additional tests,

culminating in a major operation for removal of my spleen. There had not been enough information to determine my chances for survival.

THE SEVENTEEN DAYS from the cancer diagnosis until I entered the hospital was a period of frantic activity, during which I tried to get all my affairs in order and solve all my problems. During that time I published a cover story on Cesar Chavez in *The New Republic*, submitted a children's-book proposal to Harper & Row, worked on the article for *The Washingtonian* magazine, spent a week manning a booth at an art fair (for forty dollars a day), worked on my agriculture book, made a pathetic attempt to apply for life insurance naming Laura as beneficiary, and flew to New York to begin a $175-a-day consultancy on sugar prices. I went to three parties, several working lunches, interviewed the head of the Agricultural Stabilization and Conservation Service, advised a friend to work for Jimmy Carter's campaign, and was mentioned in Washington's newly fashionable gossip column, "The Ear." I also learned a great deal about Hodgkin's disease.

Aaron frequently observed that most patients didn't ask the detailed questions I did. He said, "Some patients want their doctors to be authoritative, omniscient. These patients want nothing to do with their doctors' logic. They want nothing to do with how the doctors think. They want to be told what to do: 'Do boom, boom, boom, and boom.' They do it. They say to themselves, 'My doctor knows about that disease. Therefore he can stop it.' Putting oneself in that position is one characteristic way of attempting to control the disease process. It's not your way, but many people do it."

Knowledge has always been my way of dealing with fear. A close friend has said about me, "You do your homework. On everything you ever do, you do your homework. You do your homework on the job and you did your homework on your disease. When I met you, I remember thinking, *Here's a man who takes everything he does seriously.* It was so amazing to me. Most people just sort of slide by and do nothing. You take notes and keep journals and letters and copies of everything and go to the library and learn about this and that. Of course, you are a writer and writers do that. But it amazed me that you did that with your illness."

Laura said, "You probe and you pick. That's the sort of stuff you do."

Aaron said, "I was the guy who had the information, who would give you the information, who would take care of you, and you leaned—almost toppled—in my direction."

Another friend pointed out, "Within a couple of weeks you had picked up enough information that you were already second-guessing him."

ON TUESDAY May 11, after driving Laura to the airport for her Puerto Rican vacation, I go to group therapy.

I have been in therapy for nearly two years—ever since the summer of 1974, when I was feeling generally dissatisfied with my life. My psychiatrist is Paul S. Weisberg. At forty-four, Paul is a sometimes-startlingly bright eclectic man from a small midwestern town who trained in law at Harvard before becoming a physician. When he considered medical school, a colleague of his father advised, "Medicine is a large house. There is room in it for anybody with a good mind." To the disapproval of his physician father, when Paul received his

M.D. from the Medical University of Wisconsin, he entered psychiatric training. After residency and a stint in the navy, Paul finally settled in Washington, where, among other things, he is Associate Clinical Professor of Psychiatry at the George Washington University School of Medicine.

Paul sees medicine as a place to synthesize new concepts and techniques and to reapply old formulations. When it was legal to do so, he received federal approval to use LSD as a therapeutic tool. He is interested in biofeedback and ESP research but is careful to separate the experimental and the unproven from established medical practice.

In 1974 I remembered meeting Paul Weisberg and liking him. I figured that seeing a shrink couldn't hurt. After having lived two years in San Francisco, being in therapy seemed no crazier than just being in California. My insurance covered much of it, and in Washington there's a certain chic about having one's psyche analyzed.

The group is also led by a second therapist, Jack Raher, a fifty-two-year-old psychiatrist from Baltimore who arrives twice weekly out of breath from what Amtrak schedules as a one-hour train ride.

Paul and Jack work well together. While I never would have begun therapy with a traditional Freudian who insists that progress be made slowly and methodically, I grow to appreciate Jack's measured counterpoint to Paul's free style, as does the rest of the group.

WHEN I BEGAN THERAPY, my *problem* was not at all clear to me. I had a good job as a newsletter editor. My work was interesting and well received by colleagues and readers. But I was dissatisfied. I could list my complaints, and some were clearly warranted. But the dissatisfaction was excessive. I was dissatisfied by the job I was doing and needlessly made things difficult for myself. I was dissatisfied with the way the office was run and became needlessly involved in self-destructive office politics. Dissatisfaction also extended to my personal life. This was before Laura, a time when I was having affairs with a stream of women, but few relationships lasted for longer than a month. The women I wanted to hold on to didn't want me. The women who wanted me I didn't want to hold on to. I argued with my parents over petty subjects, which were childish for me to fight about.

My initial attitude toward therapy was casual. I was resistant to psychiatric concepts, regarding them as somewhat silly. I wanted advice on how to get the girl, rather than an analysis of why I might be attracted to unstable or distant women. I preferred seeing Paul on an individual basis, talking to him about theology and philosophy rather than my problems. I was strongly resistant to joining a group, vying for attention with other group members, and exposing myself to the criticism of patients who didn't understand me and who were clearly worse off than I was.

AFTER ABOUT TWO YEARS, I am less skeptical. The process of therapy is interesting—unraveling why I behave the way I do and watching fellow group members make discoveries about themselves. Although I continue to remain cynical and somewhat aloof, I am becoming addicted to the twice-weekly soap opera. When will Lois see the connection between her being gang-raped at sixteen and the brittle, frequently anger-provoking way she runs her office? Will Sally acquire the self-confidence to stop letting men treat her so shabbily? How long will Frank continue to present his problems as a series of comedy one-liners? Why is Mona still preoccupied by her father's suicide when it happened over twenty years ago?

There are still times when I consider the process as a grade-B movie called *Psychoanalysis in Washington*, and when talk about the group "being like a family" and Mona's cloying insistence on hugging each of us after each session provokes uncomfortable infra dig images of encounter groups.

However, we are as intimate about our faults and fears as we are capable of being. Over time, we have begun to respect each other. The 12:30 to 2:00 Tuesday and Thursday group was at first a way-stop for people to stay a few weeks and then leave. By now, however, most of the group's nine members have been there for at least a year. Because we have invested a lot of time (and money) in working on our individual problems and helping others work on theirs, the group begins to take on its own identity. Ours is a serious, businesslike group. We care about the members but grow impatient when someone takes an unnecessarily long time to get to the point or when someone interrupts the discussion of (in group parlance, "the work of") another.

On this Tuesday, Paul is at a convention. I've just finished taking Laura to the airport. So the two people closest and most important to me, Laura and Paul, are now out of town. Even though they both have perfectly good reasons for not being there when I need them, reality doesn't prevent me from feeling abandoned.

Feeling emotionally shaky, I tell Jack and the group about the cancer diagnosis. The previous Thursday, I gave the good news about the biopsy, only to be told—on that same day—that I have Hodgkin's disease.

The group is shocked and silent.

Jack, generally successful at masking his feelings, is visibly shaken.

When I later asked what he felt, Jack said, "Subjectively I was pessimistic. I've had personal experience with it. My wife's brother died at age thirty-six—something like that—of Hodgkin's, and he went out like a light. I've had a few other situations where I've been involved with treating people. My personal experience was that it was an extremely dangerous thing to have, and I wasn't aware of what kind of treatments had evolved since that time. So I had what they call a 'guarded prognosis.' I felt badly for you."

Although he thought I would die, Jack concentrated on professional concerns. He said, "I did have the feeling that one of the issues that can contribute to any kind of disease process is the mental state. I've worked extensively in this area. It's an unknown. Where there is some alleviation of the emotional factors, that can be an important factor in how the disease process turns out. My reaction is always to work with the person to try, as far as the individual can, to minimize the damage with the unresolved conflicted feelings, particularly the feeling of helplessness and rage that one has to contend with. Especially helplessness—that can be devastating."

Jack said, "One of the impacts of your having cancer is the apparent confirmation of your lifelong feeling that you are not adequate, that there's something missing from you."

PAUL RETURNS on the same Thursday I am scheduled for the bone-marrow biopsy. I enter the 12:30 group session worrying about the pain Aaron is going to inflict. Jack, as is customary, fills Paul in on developments in his absence.

Paul goes to the bookshelf, pulls out a medical text, and

begins reading the description of Hodgkin's disease. Read aloud, it sounds especially frightening. The group members are quiet and look uncomfortable.

Paul asks cold, unemotional questions, eliciting details about what Aaron has done so far and what he plans to do. Occasionally, he fills gaps in my medical knowledge. Mostly, it seems like an extensive grilling to check the witness for command of the facts. "How do you feel?" he asks.

"The experience seems unreal. Mostly, I feel nothing—empty inside. I want to continue to feel nothing and function automatically. I don't want to think about how I feel."

"Don't you feel angry? Don't you feel like raising your fist to the heavens and shouting at God, 'Why me?' "

"I did feel like that at first. And I did feel angry at you because you weren't around when I first learned that I had cancer."

After talking about my anger at him, Paul says, "I suggest that you seriously consider the possibility that the disease might kill you, that the tests might reveal the cancer to be in a more advanced state. Even if the disease is only Stage One, you might be one of those who do not survive the odds. After all, someone has to be on the losing side of the odds. Whether you live or die, it will be a valuable experience for you. I think you should regard this as an adventure."

PAUL LATER SAID, "First of all, I didn't want to be caught in a sympathetic posture. To be sympathetic to you at the time would have been disastrous. To treat you in a classic psychoanalytic role, at that point, and just be a passive listener, would not have been in your interest, because it would have given you more than enough opportunity to build up a big case about how terrible things were for poor Joel. It was important to be very clear and focus primarily on the reality of the situation.

"The fear attached to the surgery and the fear attached to whatever was about to happen were bound to be substantial. One way of reducing those fears was to manage them like an engineer, that is, to think in terms of numbers and in terms of probabilities of outcome—to dry it out, take the juice out. So I went into the possibility of death in a kind of humdrum tone of voice—I was drying it out for you as much as possible—in order to alleviate the lurking-monster stuff that goes along with the treatments for cancer. We go to this step. We go to that step. And then we do that."

IN THE THREE group sessions remaining before my entry into the hospital, I talk about death, and curiously it is a relief. Death helps prepare a map for the kind of journey I'm on. I am in the early stages of treatment for a fatal disease. If the treatment fails, then the road to death will be relatively short. If the treatment succeeds, then the road to death can be long, stretching the average expected lifespan of a twenty-eight-year-old man. Where I am—as with all living creatures—is unknown. The difference between me and everyone else is the Hodgkin's disease, which suddenly and unexpectedly makes death a matter of immediate concern.

However, it is difficult for a healthy twenty-eight-year-old man to have a reference point for considering death. Generally death and debilitation are realities the aged face as their peers experience it. For young men and women, death is something they will eventually have to consider, but they don't think about it much because they assume—generally correctly—that death is far off in the distant future, many decades away. Unlike my peers and unlike the aged, I suddenly and unexpectedly have to consider the possibility of premature death and premature debilitation.

PAUL LATER SAID, "One point of focusing on the possibility of death was to begin a process whereby you could actualize, you could validate the existence that you have had. This was instead of feeling like you were among the nonbeing—the way you frequently felt in your childhood. So to talk about death as an ending, to talk about death as a natural finalization of a life that has been real, had the net effect of actualizing for you, of allowing you to feel that you exist. When you contrast what may be the eventual outcome with what is, then you strengthen the focus on what is. You actualize what is."

Another reason for the death talk was to begin preparations in case I did die or was sick for long periods of time. Paul was afraid that if the results of my hospitalization were not good, if I was unexpectedly confronted with news that was inconclusive or grim, then I would tune out both him and everyone else. He was afraid that the anger and helplessness I'd feel would be so pervasive and so depressing that I'd hide, go off in a flurry of frantic activity, or run away to San Francisco or Rio for one last fling, screwing lots of women, taking lots of drugs. If he was going to reach me at all, then the time to do it was before the hospital, when I was still willing to listen.

He said, "I was interested in dealing with the poignancy, that your life might end prematurely and that you might be left with a lot of things that you hadn't done yet. One of the preparations was to help you grieve, if such were necessary, for the residual disability or death that could result from your having cancer.

"I worked at helping you go through the grieving process for the life that you wouldn't complete, the course of things that you would not finish in the normative manner. The value is that when somebody has gone through the grieving process and experienced the anger, experienced the rage, the detachment, and then the resolution, then there is a sense of wholeness about the person. You see it a whole lot with people who have cancers they do die of, but they have a year to process it. They go through a real identifiable grieving process. Those who are able to finish it and be resolved are able to die with a sense of self rather than a sense of being fractioned, of being cut up into pieces, of not being able to put it together."

The group, Paul noted, was helpful because the members were able to give me emotional support. "If I didn't have the group to rely on," he said, "I would have had to have been more emotional, and that would have diminished my effectiveness."

ALL OF THIS is very intense. As I go from one group session to the next the intensity gets heavier, like an enormous weight. On Thursday, May 20, at the end of the last group session before the hospital, I cry. It is the first time in years that I've cried. It is the first time the group has ever seen me cry. "The crying," Paul says, "is a good thing. It means that you acknowledge your fear and are willing to forgive yourself for it."

DORIS IS A disaster relief specialist for the federal government. She is a chunky, attractive blond in her mid-twenties who comes from a small town in Pennsylvania where unemployment is high, religious and ethnic traditions are fixed, and girls are supposed to live with their parents until they have a church wedding and marry someone of the same nationality. She is the second of three girls. Doris discovered that leaving home for a career in Washington was a major undertaking. She felt that her independent course made her a "tainted woman." While her intelligence and ambition made it impossible to stay in Pennsylvania, her attachment to parents and tradition left her feeling guilty. Doris is a devout woman who attends church regularly, and she became very close to her priest. The priest tried to reassure her that the church did not require her guilt and her excessive confessions for petty sins. Finally he recommended that she see Paul.

Paul established a reputation for using group therapy for patients traditionally treated on an individual basis. Paul's groups mixed patients from different backgrounds who had a broad range of emotional problems. Doris described her reaction to the suggestion that she join a group: "I remember thinking, *No thank you. I'll just have private sessions.*" She said, "I was afraid of the crazies that I would meet. Having been persuaded to join, I remember thinking that some of them were really outlandish and wondered what I was doing there. *These people are really out of my league. I'm just upset, but they're crazy.*" At other times, Doris said, she felt intimidated by those of us who were less openly "crazy." She complained that she didn't understand Paul's multisyllabic words and literary allusions and was unable to follow Jack's complicated formulations. She complained that she wasn't smart enough for the group and didn't have the "guts" to communicate honestly with her parents the way some members did.

There are times when I felt really close to Doris because we both came from religious backgrounds with strictly defined boundaries. I admire her simplicity and emotional honesty.

There is no pretense to her feelings, and she doesn't need (as I often do) to hide behind a contrived persona. Earlier that year, her father died of cancer, and I was moved by her devotion to him and by the dogged way she went about holding on to the best in him.

When I told the group about the cancer, Doris said, "I remember thinking that if he could die, I could die. And if he did die, this world was a really fragile place." She said, "For the first time I thought of the group as a family. We were all really concerned about you, and we began rallying around to try to help you, the way you do when a family member gets sick."

Doris said that when Paul and I discussed the statistics, "I couldn't believe how cold and unemotional Paul was—in fact, how cold and unemotional you both were."

At first, she said, "I remember thinking, *Boy, for being really sick, he has got all the causes and effects and all the intellectual notions about this disease and this sickness in his head to a T, and I don't know how he can do that. I'd be distraught, and he's acting intellectually about it.*' I didn't understand how you could do that at all."

Doris's experience with her father made her suspicious of intellectualization. "I was really concerned, because the thought of somebody I knew—not a father, not a friend, or somebody I really expected to die—being susceptible to serious sickness really upset me.

"No, I didn't have the feeling that you would die. But I also didn't have the feeling that you would be well. I had the feeling that the cancer wouldn't all be removed the first time and you'd have to keep going back to the hospital. I didn't have much faith in the kind of cure you were talking about. I really didn't. So that stuff that Paul was doing with the statistics and so on—I didn't believe a word of it."

Then, she said, "Toward the end you were acting really sad—controlled, but sad. One or two sessions before you went into the operation, you lost your feistiness. You're a feisty, exuberant person. But right before you went in, I think you lost your feistiness. I remember thinking, *He doesn't have a very good attitude about going into the hospital.* I guess I must have been thinking about my father, because my father refused to acknowledge that he was sick. They didn't tell him he had cancer. His attitude was *Oh, I'm going to be out of this place pretty soon, and when I get back* . . . , which was a whole mask for probably knowing he was going to die. And I remember thinking, *Well, Joel has got it all down, and he's probably got it written someplace all the possible things that could happen, all the possible things that could go wrong.* Then when you got sad about going to the hospital, I wondered whether you thought you'd ever get out."

SALLY, who is a year younger than I, is a fund raiser. She is a petite brunette with good taste in clothes and is well read. On weekends she goes on elaborate hiking expeditions in the West Virginia mountains. She is Jewish, her father is a dentist, and she was raised in upstate New York. She is the eldest of two children and hated the attention lavished on her brother.

Her mother had told her, "Sally, you're such a bad girl that after you I don't want any more children." Despite her brother's later birth, the comment stayed with Sally for years. She felt required to make a perpetually losing attempt to win her mother's love—especially inappropriate behavior for an adult living hundreds of miles from home.

When she first came into therapy, Sally had difficulty holding on to a job. She had trouble relating to older women in positions of authority. Gradually, she is making steady progress toward establishing a secure career and enjoying life without the depression that comes whenever she feels pleasure.

Sally commented, "One of the biggest things I had to deal with when I first came to group was, *This doesn't mean I'm crazy, that I'm sick, that I can't handle things.* On one level I know that you don't have to be nutty, sick, whatever to be in group. On the other hand, inside I felt like there was something really wrong or inadequate that I couldn't live my life and do it 'right'—whatever that is—by myself."

At first, Sally and I took an instant dislike toward each other. The day I entered group, I described my wish that therapy would help free me from my emotions so I could live in a more efficient and logical manner. Reminded of a series of unfeeling boyfriends, she said, "You should get in touch with your emotions and learn to trust them."

I said angrily, "That's a lot of hackneyed nonsense, and you know it."

She reminded me of the worst qualities in my former wife—the whining and dependency. I reminded her of her brother. Because of me, she felt she wasn't getting enough of Paul's and the group's attention. When she discussed an intimate problem, I closed in on her, asking relevant questions in a harsh tone. Frequently, she responded by crying, to which I responded by anger. Slowly, the worst of our fighting began to abate. We began to develop respect and affection for each other.

Referring to the time when I told of my cancer, Sally

said, "I remember the whole group having a feeling of shock or surprise, particularly since several days before you had said it was nothing. We had all relaxed. Now there was a lot of real concern, a lot of sadness."

She said, "You know, I always have the feeling that it will never happen to me. So it made it more real to me. I thought a lot about how I would have reacted in your situation. I don't think I would have handled it as well. I tended to feel that I'd just be reduced to a mass of quivering jelly."

Sally said that at first she didn't think I would die. "I mean there were times later on when I certainly thought that was a possibility for you, feared for you that it might be a possibility. But I think when you first hear about cancer, you don't focus on what the consequences are quite that quickly. You focus on a lot of the fears surrounding the bad press cancer has had. I mean it's just associated with a whole lot of pain and trauma—psychological pain, too.

"I thought a lot about my own mortality. You were the first person I knew who had cancer, except for relatives I wasn't close to. Particularly, you were the first person who was my age. That was a real shocker. Prior to that, cancer was always something that older people got. A different generation was supposed to get it. The fact that you were the first person I knew and we were so close in age made it seem more like a reality instead of some vague dark cloud out there. So, it made it more immediate—something that could happen to me."

IN PREPARING for the hospital, I ask Aaron to call Paul so they both know what is going on. Aaron says you have to be crazy to see a psychiatrist and "You're not crazy." Nevertheless, Aaron calls. I also set up a private session so Laura, Paul, and I can talk about me. I feel lucky, not only because my physician is competent, but also because Laura loves me and because I have two good shrinks and a group to lean on. I want my medical team to coordinate with my "emotional support team." I make sure that it happens.

WHEN AARON talked to Paul, he wanted to know how serious the risk of depression was. "What did you tell him?" I later asked. Paul said, "I told him the risk of depression was considerable."

LAURA RETURNS from Puerto Rico on Sunday, May 16. The tests Aaron keeps ordering require forms, asking for my "closest relative." I want to put down Laura's name. "If anyone is going to be responsible for me and take care of me, I want you to do it."

She agrees, asking, "Do you want your mother involved at all?"

"No."

I don't have to explain. She understands.

"Have you told her you have cancer?"

"No."

"Are you going to tell her?"

"I haven't decided yet, but I don't think so."

She doesn't understand that, but she makes no comment.

I describe to Laura a conversation I had with my agent, Fran. Her husband, Robert, developed brain cancer while they were living together just before their marriage. She told me that at the hospital the family so mobbed the physicians that they clammed up and stopped giving information to anyone. "You'll find out more and you'll get more honest information if the doctor knows that he only has to tell it once rather than twenty or thirty times," Fran advised. That seemed reasonable. Fran said, "Since I didn't have any formal status, since I wasn't *married* to Robert, I had a hard time getting any information at all."

I say to Laura, "I don't want to shut you out. I love you and trust you. When I am in the hospital I want you to be the only spokesman for my condition. I don't want my doctors talking to anyone else but you. You can relay information to everyone else."

She says, "Your mother is not going to like that."

"I don't care. Will you do it?"

"Yes."

I arrange for Laura to meet with Aaron. Aaron has angered me by refusing to let me meet Hodgkin's disease patients who've survived, saying, "I think there's a problem with confidentiality." However, he is gracious about briefing others on my condition. "If your parents or anyone else wants to talk to me," he offers, "I'll be glad to tell them what I know. It might reassure them."

I explain to Aaron how important Laura is to me, that I want him to describe to her the staging and treatment process and the probability of my survival. "Laura has agreed to be my spokesman when I'm in the hospital." Aaron agrees to inform his associates and Dr. Simpson and *his* associate of Laura's status and says, "I'll be delighted to talk to her."

After their appointment together, I talk to Laura. "How did it go?"

"Fine."

"Did he reassure you?"

"Yes."

"Do you like him?"

"He's okay."

"What do you mean, 'He's okay'? Don't you like him?" I'm concerned about her tone and her brief, businesslike response.

"Look, he's your doctor. He's a little young, and he's conceited, but he seems to know what he's talking about. Also, you trust him and that's important. I don't have to be thrilled with him. All I have to do is talk to him. Okay?"

"Do you have any problem talking to him, getting information out of him?"

"No."

I decide to leave the subject alone. Laura has been moody since her return from Puerto Rico. I've been moody too. The rhythms of our individual moodiness are poorly timed. When she's up, I'm down, and vice versa. Talking about substantive matters makes us both testy. So we avoid the serious by drinking too much, making fun of people we know, holding each other a lot. I decide that Laura needs some time to work through her feelings. I certainly do. We both are extremely busy. The week before I enter the hospital, Laura starts her new job. I have deadlines to meet. Despite her tone, I am pleased about Laura's appointment with Aaron. I feel fortunate that I have a competent physician, that I have Laura's love, and that Aaron, who will treat my disease, and Laura, who will give me emotional support, are working together.

YEARS LATER, Laura elaborated on her feelings about the interview with Aaron. "I didn't set up the interview anyway. You did. I didn't like that very much, but I did a lot of things because I wanted to do what would make you feel good. You seemed to want me to see him. I felt awkward because I wasn't sure why I was there.

"I thought he had a very condescending attitude toward me. I assumed he knew what he was talking about—sort of. I mean he's a doctor and a specialist and he said you could live a normal lifespan. I had to believe him a little bit because I'm not a real expert, but I was skeptical. I mean cancer is cancer to me. I didn't like him anyhow, so that probably didn't help. He was pompous and he talked about the difference in our ages, yours and mine, which I thought was totally irrelevant to the issue. I think he felt that I didn't really have a position to ask him about your situation. That is to say, I wasn't your wife and I wasn't your mother and I wasn't related to you. So his attitude was, *What business do you have being concerned about Joel?* He asked me, 'Don't you think you're too old for Joel?' I was pissed."

After I was in the hospital, but before Laura had told me any of this, it was clear that there was hostility between her and Aaron. I had somehow failed to make it clear to Laura exactly why I set up the interview with Aaron in the first place. But she didn't tell me about her misgivings or about her feelings that Aaron had acted in an "immature" way. Aaron later said that his recollection of the interview was very different from hers. "I never would have acted in such a meddling way. It would have been completely inappropriate." Whatever actually happened, Laura didn't tell me there was a problem while I still could have done something about it. Afterward, she explained, "I didn't want to undermine your confidence in your doctor." As a result, the woman who gave me love, who gave me the emotional support that helped me through my difficulties, didn't tell me about her feelings. The physician whose competence produced a timely diagnosis and helped save my life proved incapable of securing Laura's trust in him—a trust I needed her to have.

Years later, I interviewed Aaron for his impressions of my behavior following the cancer diagnosis. "This is going to sound like an evasion," Aaron said, "but I don't believe it is fair for any human being to make a value judgment about how somebody else feels when gutsy questions arise of that person's mortality and frailty. I think the threat of death is an ultimate organic shock. I don't think there is any shock that is more elemental to a living organism than the threat of its own death. And to stand in judgment about how somebody responds to the threat of his own death is something that is beyond me. So, when you ask me do I think you adjusted well to it, reacted well to it, I don't have an answer. I don't know. I don't formulate things in those terms.

"What the hell do you care what I think about how you reacted? I think a meaningful question for you to ask is not, Did I, Joel Solkoff, react well? That's a dumb question. A sensible question would be, When I reacted the way I did, did I get help where I needed it, when I needed it? You should be judging how I reacted to your reaction, not the other way around."

ON WEDNESDAY, May 19, at 12:30 in the afternoon, I have a liver-spleen scan. An isotope is injected painlessly into my arm. Acting as a radioactive dye, the isotope reaches my liver and spleen, where it begins beaming out rays. As I lie on a table surrounded by impressive machinery, a scanner picks up the rays and broadcasts them onto a screen. Turning to the side, I can see my liver and spleen on television.

This test emphasizes another dimension of the cancer experience. It is interesting. The technology can do fantastic things. I am fascinated by machinery that makes it possible to *see* the internal workings of my body.

I suspect that one reason patients insist on boring listeners with operation stories is because of this peculiar sense of excitement. Not only do medical procedures make one feel self-important, but the more sophisticated and less painful they become, the more one has a feeling of participating in and appreciating a strange new dimension of self-discovery.

The scan serves as a surgical aid to Simpson. He now knows that neither the liver nor the spleen is grossly enlarged. If either were, that might cause problems during the operation.

MY BOOK, *You Reap What You Sow: America Without an Agriculture Policy*, is finally beginning to take shape. Some friends have steered me to consultancy jobs, which will earn me enough money to finish the book without compromising journalistic objectivity. I am an ambitious, self-indulgent young man who has more energy than he knows what to do with and who has trouble organizing his life and exercising self-discipline. I know all that. But I am finally beginning to untangle the complications of my career and finances. I don't need this damn cancer. If I have to put up with it at all, then it will have to fit into my schedule, which is very tight.

Aaron and I are constantly arguing about when the next test will be held. Finally, he says, "I've had it. I'm your doctor. No more delays."

We compromise. I convince him that business prevents me from entering the hospital next Monday morning. I have to go to New York for the day. He schedules me for admission on Tuesday morning at 9:00 A.M.

8

On the morning of the nineteenth, before my liver-spleen scan, I finally call my mother. I am feeling shaky about the whole idea of surgery and hospitals. I want Mother to respect my wishes for my treatment and care during my illness. I realize that telling her will mean that she'll want to see me. She is, after all, my mother.

However, tomorrow, I have a final appointment with Aaron before entering the hospital. On Friday, I have an interview with the director of the USDA agency that administers price-support programs. During the weekend, I want to be alone with Laura. On Monday, I have to work as a consultant on sugar prices. On Tuesday, I am scheduled to enter the hospital for tests before next Thursday's operation.

I don't want to see Mother at all. I worry that if we see each other we'll fight about Laura—her religion, age, children. I don't want to fight with anyone about anything. I decide that

I can handle seeing Mother after the operation, after one or two days have gone by and I've had time to recover from surgery. Then she can fly home to Florida reassured that I am all right. End of mother problem.

Although I am not feeling kindly toward Mother when I begin the phone call, my feelings quickly change. She is my mother. Despite everything, I love her. I know that it is painful to learn that her son has cancer and might die from it. I say, "Mother, I have a serious disease."

"What is it?"

"It's a form of cancer called Hodgkin's disease."

"Yes, that is a serious disease." Each word is said slowly, with intense seriousness. She is sad and she loves me. She loves me despite our differences.

Then, suddenly, she dismisses my illness as if it were inconsequential. "Of course, you'll be all right." She begins talking about God. "Nothing really serious can ever happen to my son." I react automatically—the way I did as a child when she dismissed something I regarded as important. I become angry and withdrawn, no longer attempting to assure her, coldly stating the unpleasant. "This disease can kill me," I tell her.

"Don't be ridiculous," she says. "You won't die. You can't. You're my son." Then she says, "Why did this happen to me?" (as if she has the disease). She repeats, "Why did this happen to me right now? It couldn't have come at a worse time."

She wants to come up instantly: "I will call my office, have someone take over my schedule, get the next plane up, and move into your apartment to take care of you."

"No one," I say, "is going to set foot in my apartment." Five days before entering the hospital is not a good time for a thorough housecleaning. I know that if I let Mother or any other relative into the apartment, the apartment will be cleaned in my absence and I'll hear in detail how filthy it was and how difficult it was to clean.

Mother says, "Who's going to take care of you?"

"Laura."

Ignoring me, she says, "Well, if you don't want me to take care of you, I'll ask my mother and your father to come up and take care of you. They can move into your apartment. My mother can clean and cook and your father can be there for moral support."

I say, "No one is taking care of me. I don't want you to take care of me. I don't want my grandmother taking care of me. I don't want my father taking care of me. If anyone has to take care of me, Laura will. And no one is going to set foot in my apartment."

"Then where am I going to stay?" The tone implies that I am condemning her to spend long winter nights in a pup tent in Siberia. I remind her that there are hotels and that she has relatives in the area. She wants a recommendation for a hotel close to the hospital.

"Call Laura. She's an administrative assistant. It's her job to be familiar with downtown hotels and their prices."

Giving Mother Aaron's telephone number, I say, "You're welcome to talk to him. In fact, it will probably reassure you if you do. However, after I enter the hospital, I don't want more than one person asking the doctors about my medical condition. So while I'm in there, Laura has agreed to be the spokesman on my medical condition." I give her Laura's phone numbers, saying that she will be pleased to talk to the family at work or at home, if she cannot be reached at the hospital.

LOOKING BACK, Mother remembered my call. "The phone rang as I was pouring water from the teakettle. I was so glad to hear your voice. You said, 'Are you sitting down?'

"I said, 'No, I'm making a cup of coffee.'

" 'Sit down, I have something to tell you that will be very painful for you.'

" 'Okay,' said I, 'I'm sitting.' Of course my thoughts were on another subject completely. [She thought I had married Laura.] Then came your words about your illness. I sat there transfixed. It wasn't at all what I had expected to hear. As you spoke and gave me all the details of how you discovered the lump, through the details of the diagnosis of Hodgkin's, I began jotting down all the things you said.

"I tried to comment as best I could under the circumstances. I tried to be optimistic and you countered with, 'I don't want to hear any of your faith in God [she used the Hebrew word] or anything like that. Nor do I want to see you at all until the surgery is over. Do not try to see me before the operation. I will be very angry if you come. You may come and see me when the anesthesia wears off, not before. Everything will be handled through Laura, nothing through you, et cetera, et cetera, et cetera.'

"The first thing I did when you hung up was to call your doctor. He was very encouraging and reassuring that the outcome would be a good one, because they caught it early or to quote his words, 'It was in a lollipop state.' Knowing the facts, I was armed for what was ahead. In my heart I knew no serious harm would come to you and that your chances for complete recovery were excellent.

"I was in a quandary. I certainly didn't want to antagonize you in any way. You were so angry at me for my stand on other matters, and now you were angry with your illness. The two didn't go together, but you decided that I was not to be part of this to help you in any way. It puzzled me. *Why did he call if he didn't want me there? Was it only to hurt me and to make me feel guilty?* If you didn't want me, why did you call me?

"It was hard for me to swallow the hurt of your rejection. I, who had spent so many years of my life with you as its pivotal figure. There wasn't anything I had that I didn't give you as a child. I gave you more than material things. I gave of myself. It wasn't easy to do, but there wasn't anything I would do if I knew it would be harmful to you. I tried to make a good home life for you and to give you a good life so that you would grow up and be a whole person. I did this at a time when being a single parent was not exactly the in thing. I always thought we had a beautiful relationship when you were growing up, and I prided myself on that. But I was a person in my own right, too, and my ideals were not the kinds of things I could compromise. My people came before me, personally. Turning my back on the future of the Jewish people was nothing I could ever condone.

"I wanted to be loving to you as I had been in the past and do all I could, but I was being blocked. You were my son for twenty-eight years, and a relationship that was relatively new—yours and Laura's—was going to destroy everything our family could do. We were shut out, and I was scared. Scared, maybe, that the great faith I had would not come through as I wanted it to. Maybe something would not go well. Then what? I was your mother. I had to be there. We were your family, and I was very hurt."

She continued, "I had to reroute my entire schedule because I was supposed to have closing exercises at school. I called Laura and told her what my plans were. I asked her to please not tell you that I would be there in the waiting room all day Thursday because I did not want to upset you."

HAVING TOLD MOTHER, I am in a rush to tell my father. I feel as I did in childhood, trying to give each of my parents equal time, loyalty, and love. I want to make sure that Dad hears about my disease from me—before Mother has a chance to call him. Although Mother and Father rarely talk to each other, I know this will be one of the exceptions.

Reaching him is not easy. He is not in all Wednesday morning, afternoon, or evening, either at the office or at home. The following morning I call at 8:00 A.M. I want to catch him before he leaves for work. Dad is not a morning person and I generally avoid talking to him then.

Billie, my stepmother, answers the phone. "What's wrong?" Obviously something is wrong or why am I calling so early?

I say, "Let me talk to my father," trying to be friendly, while evading the question. It is an impossible situation. I am stiff and formal, as I have never been with Billie.

She understands that whatever is wrong, I want to tell Dad before telling her. She puts him on.

He sounds terrible. He is groggy. His voice is full of phlegm. He obviously hasn't had his first cup of coffee. My father is an old man. He is seventy-four—twenty-three years older than my mother. However, he looks and acts decades younger than he is. That morning he sounds old and acts old. I feel like a jerk for waking him up with news I've been keeping from him for weeks. What is the rush? Why do I have to tell him this terrible news? Why is the timing so rotten? Already I have made the situation more dramatic than I want it to be, and I haven't even started talking.

I tell him that I have a form of cancer called Hodgkin's disease, that I will probably be cured, and that I am entering the hospital in five days for exploratory surgery. "You are welcome to call my doctor who will describe the disease to you."

He doesn't want the number. "I'll talk to your mother. She can call your doctor and tell me what he says. Have you told your mother?"

"I told her yesterday. I tried calling you all day yesterday but you weren't in."

He says, "I don't want you unduly upsetting your mother." Dad listens to my not wanting anyone to visit me until after the operation. "That's all right with me. I'm very busy now and don't have time to take the trip. Anyway, I think it's more appropriate that your mother visit you, and it will be awkward if both of us visit at the same time." Reluctantly, he writes down Laura's phone numbers.

His stepdaughter, Susan, lives in nearby Reston. "I'll ask Susan to come to the hospital to visit you. She'll be my representative," he says.

BILLIE LATER told me that when Dad hung up, "He wept like a baby." He and I had a few telephone conversations after that. However, Dad didn't get the chance to visit me until over a year later.

ON MONDAY MORNING, May 24, the day before entering the hospital, I'm on the Eastern Airlines Washington–New York shuttle. My shirt feels tight around my neck. I keep massaging the skin on my neck and chin, thinking that I'm getting fat and must go on a diet. "After I get out of the hospital," I tell myself, thinking about the difficulties of eating less. I also promise myself to begin exercising regularly, thinking distastefully about jogging and calisthenics. The hospital reminds me that I don't want to think about the hospital. At all. Period. This is going to be a long day, and I want to enjoy the idea of being a well-paid consultant, flying to New York and back on the same day.

I worry about whether my shirt is too flashy for a New York law firm. Laura lent me her briefcase (green, to match her eyes) bought on an expensive impulse at Camalier & Buckley. The leather briefcase is beautiful, although perhaps a little too green for New York. I worry about the color and then worry about Laura. She has been back nearly a week, looking marvelous because her sunburn has turned tan. I think about marrying her, about being a father to her children, about how much I love her.

It seems strange that I'm not interested in having sex with other women. The intensity and electricity between Laura and me is frequently frightening and uncontrollable, but it is always pleasurable. Always. Last night was no exception. In fact, we made love with even more fury than usual. But after it was over I felt sad and distant.

Aaron said that if I am given radiation treatment, it will probably make me impotent for a while. I have never been impotent. The idea frightens me. If Laura and I are unable to have sex, will she leave me? Will I really have to give up sex? Is it possible that something could make me uninterested in sex? How could that happen?

I turn to the commodity column in the *Times* and begin

reading. I read the same sentence over and over. I decide instead to concentrate on the spot price of sugar, unable to remember the number for more than a second. I stare out the window, watching the clouds and thinking, "This may be my last trip anywhere."

The cab deposits me at 120 Broadway. Too early for the appointment, I walk down the block to Trinity Church thinking about how exciting New York is and regretting that I've left it. I decide against looking at the tombstones in the churchyard and instead walk back up Broadway to the massive Equitable Building where James R. Truman of the law firm of Rutherford, Hamm & Benning is scheduled to meet me at 9:00 A.M.

The thirtieth-floor receptionist brings a cup of coffee with sugar and cream. Meanwhile Truman comes down from the thirty-first floor. We meet in a large conference room, littered with used Styrofoam cups from a previous meeting. I like Truman. He is bright and quick—friendly in a cool, professional way. We quickly get down to business.

Truman specializes in admiralty law. His client owns a ship whose cargo of sugar was damaged at sea and had to be dumped overboard. That happened in 1974, when the price was very high. Truman wants evidence that the sugar market was rigged and the high price was artificial. He explains the rules of admissible evidence. While I suspect USDA officials and commodity speculators of engaging in shady practices, I tell him that proof might be difficult. I explain how the price of sugar was determined in 1974, why the U.S. price was different from the so-called world price and the relevance of these prices to his client.

I am tired and preoccupied. But the consultancy excites

me. I know there has been high-level skulduggery in both government and business. I know where to look, and I will be paid very well for looking. It seems like fun. I tell Truman that I can't begin until I "complete another assignment in two weeks." (I am pleased with my use of the word "assignment.") He says that is fine and asks me to get him some government reports in the interim.

We lunch at the Downtown Athletic Club, watching the harbor traffic. He talks animatedly about the Tall Ships scheduled to arrive for the Bicentennial. I have trouble thinking about the Bicentennial. If the operation results are bad, will I be dying in two months?

After returning to Washington, I meet Laura for a late supper at the Hay-Adams Hotel. The massive dining room is empty. We sit on enormous wingback chairs next to the dormant fireplace, drinking Korbel Brut's special Bicentennial champagne. During coffee, Laura decides to move over to my chair and sit on my lap. It is a drunk, melancholy evening. We start necking in the restaurant. A matronly hostess gives us a stern lecture on decorum. Laura gets furious, threatening to complain to the manager. I try to calm her down, not willing to make a fuss.

Laura says, "I'm feeling guilty about not spending enough time with the kids. Why don't we spend the night at my house?" Instead, Laura comes over to my apartment. She doesn't want to be alone that night and she doesn't want me to be alone. I tell her that I want to make love, then I want to be alone to pack for the hospital. She says, "I won't argue with you. I'll do what you want."

I AM TIRED. It has been a long day. I wash the dishes and set out my clothes for the following morning. That night I shower and even shave. I clip my fingernails, then my toenails. The nail on the large toe of my left foot looks ingrown. I become obsessed with it, using several pairs of scissors, hacking away at the nail and drawing blood. Finally, I give up. I figure that an ingrown toenail is the least of my worries.

9

GEORGE WASHINGTON UNIVERSITY HOSPITAL dominates Washington Circle. The circle—originally designed with carriages in mind—is now a confusing traffic jam along the outside and a small well-kept park on the inside. The park has flowers, an occasional bum, and the obligatory bronze statue. The statue was unveiled in 1860 and intended to show an "undaunted" George Washington riding a terrified horse past exploding cannonballs and into enemy lines. Today the expression on Washington's face has been obliterated by dirt and pigeon droppings. The horse, however, still looks scared—nostrils flaring and eyes bulging.

The hospital's principal architectural value is its convenient location—six blocks from the White House and a short walk from the area's professional office buildings where, among others, my internist and surgeon practice. Ambulances careen around the circle and into the hospital's modern driveway. Buses stop directly in front of the Twenty-second Street entrance.

The hospital, however, is not located conveniently to where I live. Capitol Hill is on the other side of town; the bus routes are complicated; the subway is under construction; cabs avoid the Hill. The easiest way to get there is to ride my red Tigre America bicycle (made in Taiwan). Although it is crazy to ride a bicycle to an operation, on Tuesday morning I waste half an hour considering the logistics of bicycling. Finally, I call for a Diamond Cab.

I don't know what to pack, so I bring pens and notebooks. I also arrive with a manual on commodity-future trading, a compilation of agriculture department regulations, *Congressional Staff Directory*, the *I Ching* (a relic from San Francisco hippy days), a Bible, and a White House study on sugar prices.

At 9:00 A.M. I stride through the hospital door, eager to finish with the unpleasant business as quickly as possible. I am overwhelmed by the nauseating odor. Disinfectant does a poor job of masking what smells like old shoes and pus. Meanwhile it is difficult to find the admissions office. The hospital is being "modernized." The principal entrance was blocked by scaffolding. I learn that the door I came through is a side door. I am on the wrong floor. On the right floor, I again ask professionals, identifiable by name tags and lab coats, but the directions vary. The office has been moved several times during the continual construction.

I am afraid of forms, and the pile before me looks especially intimidating. The lady behind the desk is friendly, helping me get through the paperwork quickly. "All done," she says and smiles. "Now I'll call for a wheelchair, and you'll be in your room shortly."

"I don't need a wheelchair. I'm perfectly capable of walking."

A hospital rule requires, she explains, that in order for inpatients to travel within the building, they must be pushed in a wheelchair or on a gurney by authorized personnel.

"That's ridiculous."

She's not about to argue. Twenty minutes later, an orderly arrives. He hasn't mastered the technique of maneuvering wheelchairs in and out of elevators. I keep backseat driving. The orderly ignores me. Getting from the ground floor to my sixth-floor room is excruciatingly slow. I feel humiliated by this pretense that I am incapacitated.

It does not occur to me that large institutions require established procedures to ensure that work gets done and everyone's duties are clear. My previous experience has not included bureaucratic regimen and routine—having never served in the army, government, or a large corporation. Children's hospitals have orientation sessions: "This is the admissions office. This is your room. This is your orderly. This is the nurse. These people are here to help you, but they are also here to help the other patients. They get their work assignment from . . . The rules are designed to . . . If you need help just . . ." Adults are expected to behave like adults.

I am capable of understanding that the hospital's construction, the request for my insurance card, the rule requiring that an admitted patient be escorted to his room, are not deliberate attempts to inconvenience me personally. But cancer has given me an excuse to be irrational. I might realize that my irrationality—like other forms of stupidity—is basically self-defeating if someone would tap me on the shoulder and say, "Calm down. You're only making it harder on everyone." Instead, feeling isolated and picked on, I behave like a stereotypically bad patient, acting out a Borscht Belt routine on hospital inefficiency. Irritability and impatience over trivia help mask my rational fear and anger over being sick, having an operation, and not knowing my chances of survival. Instead of worrying about that, I worry about the slow elevator ride up to the hospital room.

Room 6225S is all right. The fellow occupant is a man in his mid-forties, named Bob Langley. A Cadillac dealer from Virginia, he was admitted for tests and is reluctant to leave. "This is better than a vacation," Langley says. "I got away from the wife and got more rest here than in a Holiday Inn. I should do this more often. What are you here for?"

I tell him.

Fear becomes visible in his gray eyes. He suddenly is preoccupied by packing.

I am assigned the window bed. The closet is on Bob Langley's side. A curtain can be drawn between us, giving a form of privacy. We each have our own sinks. The bathroom is down the hall.

A nurse comes in to begin the routine. Blood pressure, temperature, lab samples. When she touches me, I try to pull away. She sticks a small needle in my arm. I scream.

"Jesus Christ," my roommate says, "it's only a blood test. Calm down."

"I can't. I'm scared."

He finishes packing and leaves.

Another nurse arrives with a series of questions for a new "Patient Profile." "This is a waste of time," she says good-naturedly. "No one's going to read the answers anyway. But I've got to do it, so we might as well get it over with.... 'What is the patient's emotional tone?' "

Automatically I say, "Pissed off," surprised at the reflex

nature of the response and my crudity in front of a stranger.

She smiles and shakes her head. *This one*, I imagine her thinking, *is a real kidder.*

I want to say, "I'm really pissed off. Really I am. I'm not joking. I'm frightened. I want to talk to someone about my fear—get some control over it." Instead, I smile back as she writes "Appropriate" in the answer blank. *No one is going to read this form anyway.*

She wants to know whether I have any special instructions.

"Yes, on the day of the operation, I don't want to have any visitors except my friend Laura Constable. My mother may try to come up early or someone else may want to see me, but I don't want to see anyone except Laura. Can you keep out the visitors I don't want?"

She says she can.

A resident named Dr. Eliot stops by to ask a series of questions. "Do you sweat a lot at night? Do you run high fevers or experience frequent chills? Do you itch a lot? Have you experienced sudden, inexplicable weight losses? Do you experience pain when you drink alcohol?"

Dr. Eliot writes in my chart, "The patient denies any fever. . . ."

I ask whether he knows anyone else who's had Hodgkin's disease.

He is eager to be helpful. "Why yes," he says. "Earlier this year we treated a woman right here on the same floor. She came in for a splenectomy, just like you."

"What happened to her? Do you know?"

He pauses, embarrassed. "She died." He adds quickly, "But she had sweats and fever, and you don't." He doesn't know any survivors. "But then, I'm only a resident. I'm sure Dr. Falk has successfully treated lots of Hodgkin's disease patients." He asks, "Do you understand what procedures you will experience while you're here in the hospital?"

"Yes, Dr. Falk has explained all that to me."

"Well, let me go over it again—just to be sure."

I know what they're going to do to me. Today, I will have a lymphangiogram. A dye will be inserted in my feet, making it possible to photograph the lymphatic system, otherwise invisible to X rays. Tomorrow, after the dye has completely spread, X rays will indicate any additional tumors. This may be useful to my surgeon for directing him to potentially suspicious sites. On Thursday morning, Dr. Simpson will cut open my belly, remove my spleen, and take samples of the liver and abdominal lymph nodes.

A secondary reason for the splenectomy is that the spleen is the primary organ of the lymphatic system. Removal is precautionary. The spleen functions as a kind of filter, and if for some reason it were to become backed up and enlarged, it might burst and spread cancer cells throughout the abdomen. One can lead a normal life without a spleen (the filtration function being taken over by the kidneys).

The primary reason for the operation is diagnostic. Pathologists will look for cancer by examining slices of the spleen and other samples. What they find will determine my stage and form of treatment.

Using his own language, Dr. Eliot repeats this explanation. I am annoyed at having to hear the explanation again. Also Dr. Eliot avoids mentioning what the operation is really about: when it is over, I will know the likelihood of staying alive.

Just before the lymphangiogram a nurse hands me an ugly off-white hospital gown, foam slippers, and a thin cotton gown, which looks like a smock. She instructs me to change out of my clothes and tells me how to put on the gown. I have already been warned that money and other valuables are not the responsibility of the hospital. The nurse suggests that I give them to her for safekeeping. Instead I hide my watch, wallet, and about forty dollars in cash in the room. The absence of clothes, money, and credit cards makes me feel as if I have lost identity. Without a watch I feel naked. Who am I without a driver's license? My new status is written on a plastic bracelet attached to my left wrist.

The nurse calls for an orderly. Fifteen minutes later, I am again being pushed—first to diagnostic X ray, then to another X-ray room elsewhere in the building, where a resident in the department of radiology describes the procedure for a lymphangiogram. He hands me Form 169, AUTHORIZATION FOR PERFORMANCE OF OPERATIONS AND OTHER PROCEDURES. I ask him to tell me his name. Dr. Byrd does (impatiently). I point out his failure to fill in the blank after "nature of the operation to be performed." He does, pressing the ball-point firmly against the clipboard. I am not making friends.

Dr. Byrd instructs me to lie face up on the X-ray table. He is not gentle as he takes a large needle and injects a Novocain-type substance between my first two toes. I scream.

"Don't move your foot," he yells. He tells the technician, "Hold down his legs."

A blue dye is injected between my toes. Repeat other foot. Then more anesthetic. After each foot is deadened, he slashes it open at the top. He injects more anesthetic. I scream again. My repeated screaming grows quieter as my voice begins to give out. I mumble a string of four-letter words, surprised by their vulgarity and by my inability to stop cursing. The intense pain is quickly replaced by the feeling that my feet are burning.

The resident inserts tubes inside the tops of my feet. "Hold still. If you move, the dye won't enter properly and we'll have to repeat the whole procedure again."

It is a long three hours. During most of it Dr. Byrd leaves me alone with the technician, who keeps telling me not to move. Occasionally, a tube is adjusted and more of the Ethiodol contrast dye is poured in. Sometimes I feel or imagine feeling the stuff going through my system. Lying there I promise myself to learn to meditate and conquer fear and pain. My feet continue to burn. I badly want someone to hold my hand. The nurse says no.

Dr. Byrd becomes friendlier while removing the tubes and sewing the tops of my feet. He obviously wants my cooperation to do something, but is slow in coming to the point. He says I will have to undergo this test every year for the rest of my life. I might, however, avoid a repeat if I am willing to take a new, totally painless, experimental test. His sewing is not painless, and I do not want to do anything that will please him or the hospital in any way. During the past three hours he has avoided most of my questions by rushing impatiently out of the room. After he answers my questions now, I finally agree to the test. Answers, I decide, are not easy to obtain in a hospital. Manipulation helps.

Again I wait for the orderly. In the waiting room, an elderly man observes my stitched feet and tells me about his lymphangiogram. "Three hours," he tells me, "are nothing. Why, with me, the tubes kept blocking up . . ." The horror story is long and detailed. I wonder whether I'll forever be meeting members of the stigmata club, taking off our socks and showing each other our scars.

Several elevators later, I am again lying on another table. My body is covered with mineral oil. A physician is rolling a hand-held electronic gadget over my belly. He says it is a sonar device, which is creating a picture of my insides on a television screen. Suddenly I understand what the phrase "teaching hospital" really means. My body is today's lecture.

"What's that stuff?" I ask, pointing to a lot of bubbles on the screen.

"Gas."

The class laughs.

I am embarrassed at having more gas than seems appropriate. But I want to know how the gadget works. The sonar device fascinates me. "Why did I have that painful lymphangiogram when this is just as good? What is it telling you? Do you see any Hodgkin's disease?" The medical school professor is not pleased by my questions. He is trying to teach his class and I am interrupting. I imagine him thinking that frogs don't talk when you dissect them.

Back at my room I am given a late lunch. A friend of mine with whom I spent several afternoons last week drinking Bloody Marys has left a note "to one of the best and the brightest" and a copy of *The Final Days*. I was delighted when I read the *Post*'s published account of Nixon asking Kissinger to get down on his knees: "He was hysterical. 'Henry,' he said, 'you are not a very orthodox Jew, and I am not an orthodox Quaker, but we need to pray.' " I am eager to read the book. Instead I make phone calls to get sugar material for James Truman in New York. Then I talk to Laura, who says she came by to visit, is sorry she missed me, and will return later that evening after feeding the kids.

So far my attempts to joke with nurses and other hospital personnel have been met by grimness. My quips and dry humor are either regarded literally (and thus misunderstood) or ignored in the frenetic rush. I sense an overbearing attitude that hospitals must be treated seriously. Fortunately, Simpson and Aaron are both in frivolous moods when they stop by for brief visits. Seeing them cheers me up and makes me feel less isolated.

A hospital volunteer comes by with a library van. I check out *Doctor Frigo* by Eric Ambler. The epigraph is eye-catching. Ambler quotes the last words of Emperor Maximilian of Mexico. Before being executed by a firing squad, the emperor turned to his cook and said, "You refused to believe it would ever come to this. You see you were wrong."

Laura arrives after dinner. She is wearing a dress! "The kids were really good and cooperative so I got away earlier than I expected. Here, I brought you some wine." We drink the contraband and I try to make love to her. After all, my roommate has checked out that morning, the nurse has just made rounds, and we are alone. Also, I am feeling desperate and anxious. This might be, I fear, my last chance ever to have sex again.

Laura is too nervous. I reach under her dress. She reaches under my gown. She pulls my hand away and continues jerking me off. It is difficult to climax. When I come close, I stretch out my feet. That pulls at my stitches and hurts. Finally. As I am mopping up, Robert knocks at the door.

Laura and I laugh nervously. We offer Robert a drink. He accepts it primly. He wants to refuse because he thinks that wine and laughter are inappropriate for hospitals. While we are drinking a new resident enters. I offer him some wine, which he accepts. Hallelujah. He says that I have to go downstairs for more X rays. Robert says in that case he'll leave. "No," I say, "we can all go down for the tests. Isn't that so?"

The resident can see no reason why not. "It'll only be for a little while, and your friends can stay in the waiting room."

So, when the orderly arrives Laura walks on one side of the wheelchair and Robert on the other. Robert is quickly explaining that he has to catch a plane to Pittsburgh to visit a priest friend who is a member of a religious order called "an Oratory." Robert says he is trying to decide whether to join the Oratory or the Jesuits. "Goodbye. See you soon." He leaves.

I ask Laura, "What's an Oratory?" "Damned if I know," she says.

ROBERT'S RELIGIOUS aspirations were apparent during the first eight years of our schooling at the Hebrew Academy, where he was class president. Our teachers tried to persuade him to become a rabbi. When he was eighteen his father died, and he seriously considered the rabbinate. After college he returned to Florida to care for his ailing mother, secretly attending mass every day en route to work. Often he went twice a day. The day Estelle died, he was baptized in the local Roman Catholic Church. Although Robert arranged for Estelle's Jewish funeral, he made sure that a mass was said for her.

I was Robert's confidant during much of his soul-searching. We discussed the divinity of Christ, the mystery of the sacrament, the laying on of hands. I was impressed by his sincerity and by his tortuous wrestling to determine whether he had priestly vocation. However, I doubted his ability to tolerate chastity and poverty. When he became interested in the (high) Episcopal Church, I was encouraged, because Episcopal priests are permitted greater latitude in their personal lives. Then about the time of my cancer diagnosis, Robert decided against Episcopalianism and was researching options for becoming a Roman priest including the Oratory, which was the Congregation of the Oratory of St. Philip Neri. Several months later, when my treatment was at its worst, Robert entered the Jesuit Novitiate of Saint Isaac Jogues in Wernersville, Pennyslvania. He wrote frequently, saying, "I pray for you." Years later, Robert said that fear of my death helped propel him toward holy orders. "You're like a brother to me. I just couldn't face another death in my family. I needed to cling to Mother Church." He said that when he visited me in the hospital, "I was paralyzed by fear. So I made sure that my visits to you were as brief as possible and that I was always late for an appointment elsewhere. And, of course, I sent my friends."

He certainly did. During the days that followed, there seemed to be a steady stream of Robert's Roman and Episcopal priests by my bedside. In my drugged state, the sea of clerical collars confused me. It certainly freaked out my Jewish mother.

THE X RAYS are quick. Laura and I linger over our goodnight kisses. I do not want to be left alone. I ring for a sleeping pill. It works.

At 1:00 A.M. I am awakened by the nurse doing night rounds. Temperature. Blood pressure. I am angry. I demand

107

another sleeping pill. Nurse's note: "Verbalized anger at being awakened by nurse's room rounds. Questioned need to be 'checked during the night to see if I'm still alive.' Night routine explained. House officer notified and repeat sleeping pill given." The nurse writes: "Anger reaction to diagnosis" and recommends "TLC, explanation, patience, encourage verbalization of feelings."

The second pill takes a long time to work. As Dr. Byrd predicted, the lymphatic dye is causing a fever. I am sweating, cold, and anxious. I begin reading *Dr. Frigo*.

The hero says, "At the moment it seems to me that the extent of my vulnerability has been suddenly and considerably increased." Indeed. Eric Ambler's heroes are victims tricked into fighting other people's battles according to rules they do not understand. They are trapped, which is how I feel.

A GROUP of medical students surrounds my bed before breakfast. The instructor begins feeling my neck, under my arms, and around my groin. He tells me to hold still. At the same time he is lecturing. He encourages a medical student to ask the traditional questions: "Do you sweat a lot, lose weight inexplicably, itch uncontrollably?" One student quietly joins the group after the lecture begins. She puts on her medical smock quickly, trying not to be noticed. "You're late," I say, intending to be cruel. She gives me a look of pure hatred as the class laughs at her.

By now the dye has circulated throughout the lymphatic system and the doctors have examined the X rays. Several dark spots show up near my lungs. Are they tumors? The doctors think so. My diagnosis changes from a tentative Stage I to a clinical Stage III. Dr. Simpson now has additional targets to sample during the operation. The news from the lymphangio-gram is bad. If the Stage III diagnosis holds, my odds of surviving until 1981, with the cancer wiped out by vigorous treatment, is 61.1 percent. If Simpson finds additional evidence of cancer, the odds could be worse.

WITHOUT TREATMENT, Hodgkin's disease forms cancerous tumors that progress through the system, taking over the spleen and an increasing number of lymph nodes. This retards the body's ability to rid itself of waste and reduces the blood's supply of infection-fighting lymphatic fluid. Meanwhile spreading tumors also take over nearby vital organs such as the liver and lungs. The patient dies from failure of a vital organ, from the body choking in its own waste, or from inability to fight infection. Death is generally not very painful, but it can be. The patient sweats profusely, itches to the core of his body, loses weight rapidly and unexpectedly, feels fatigued, has no appetite, and loses interest in staying alive. A steady low-grade fever can flare up, especially toward the end—with the patient feeling as if he is on fire. Patients who are treated and die are generally killed by the increasingly large doses of drugs which inexplicably fail to stop the cancer.

Technically, I was Aaron's patient. However, for the hospital's legal records I was Simpson's patient—I was there for surgery, and Simpson is a surgeon. They both visited me daily or sent their associates. Simpson, who is so at ease and reassuring by a patient's bedside or in an operating theater, later surprised me by his discomfort at being interviewed. He said he frequently had to tell patients they had cancer and their future was bleak. "I was relieved that if I found additional presence of cancer, Aaron would be the one to tell you about it. I was also relieved that if I found additional tumors, I would not be treating you." A radiologist or an oncologist would take over.

ON WEDNESDAY morning, I complain to the resident that the nurse awakened me the night before to perform needless rounds. He says he'll write an order requesting that I not be disturbed that night. When orderlies take a long time arriving with the wheelchair, I complain. When nurses fail to respond to the buzzer instantly, I complain. I complain about the orderlies to the nurses, about the nurses to the residents, about the residents to my doctors. The more I complain, the more difficult it is to get through the day. Slow festering resentment can be a lot more uncomfortable than an unanswered buzzer. By the end of Wednesday, I decide that my behavior has to change. Whether I want to or not, I force myself to become friendly and polite.

Both Aaron and Simpson's brief visits are a small part of a passing parade. The hospital personnel work in teams, operating on rotating schedules. Most of my day-to-day medical care is done by one of the residents or by the medical student assigned to the surgical team—under Simpson's orders. There is also a hematology team—under Aaron's orders—which has its residents and students. The nurses are part of a nursing team, supervised by a registered nurse who can call or wake up a resident physician if my medical condition requires or if I become too difficult to handle.

I am constantly being interrupted, tested, and questioned by people I haven't seen before. At first, I ask nurses, residents, technicians, orderlies, team physicians, medical students, and housekeeping personnel their names. But there are so many of them. The specialized nature of cancer care requires sophisticated tests, which means several wheelchair expeditions. I see the people operating equipment and conducting tests only briefly, and then I don't see them again.

As a writer I've always needed privacy. Suddenly I am in an environment where everything I do is subject to scrutiny. The color of my urine and the consistency of my bowels are questioned. On Wednesday, my new roommate arrives. He is an elderly man, moaning in pain. His presence destroys any hope that I'll be alone even when I am alone. The hospital routine is not my routine. I am awakened, fed, tested, questioned, moved, and visited according to the schedule and convenience of strangers. I feel disoriented and frightened.

On Wednesday night, a tall black orderly comes by with a razor to shave off the hair on my belly and around my genitals. This is preparation for tomorrow's surgery. I anxiously hold my breath when he whisks the razor underneath my testicles.

Thursday, May 27, Laura is here at 7:00 A.M. Her presence fills the room. I can feel her love. The injection of Demerol makes me euphoric. As I look at Laura, standing by my bedside holding my hand, no other reality exists. My body is placed on a stretcher and we are still holding hands. A voice says, "It is time for the operation."

My voice says, "I don't care as long as Laura is with me."

The stretcher moves forward. I turn to the source of the movement, and there is an orderly pushing. I turn back to Laura, squeezing her hand. We are in the corridor. I am squeezing her hand and we are in front of surgery.

The orderly says, "You have to let go of her hand now."

"No."

I look up and there is Simpson down the hallway, past the

swinging doors, dressed in his silly surgical astronaut suit. "There's Dr. Simpson," I say and smile. "Can I kiss her good-bye?" I yell.

In a faraway voice, he says, "Of course."

There is the kiss and her face. There is a quick ride forward. A man takes a needle to my arm. I turn to Simpson and try saying, "This feels wonderful." The Pentothal puts me to sleep before I can finish the sentence.

10

"WITH THE PATIENT in the supine position," Simpson dictates as he works, "under adequate anesthesia, the abdomen is prepped and draped in the usual sterile manner. A midline skin incision is then made extending from the xiphoid process to well below the umbilicus, carried down through skin and subcutaneous tissue to the level of the midline fascia, which is then opened, and the abdominal cavity is entered in the usual fashion. Exploration of the abdominal cavity is unremarkable.... Having removed the spleen, a tape is placed in the left upper quadrant. Attention is then turned to the left lobe of the liver where a wedge biopsy is done. . . ."

Tuesday's test showed dark areas at the base of my lungs—probably cancerous tumors. Today's operation, two days later, indicates that the lymphangiogram is wrong. Simpson finds no tumors. My spleen is normal. My liver is uninfected. The cancer has not reached my abdomen.

Two hours later, I am lying in the recovery room. I open

my eyes and everything seems white and swimming. Paul, my psychiatrist, is standing over my stretcher. He seems very tall, dominating the room. It is the first time I have seen him outside his office. It is the first time I've seen him wear a tie. He has a large smile. He says, "You're all right."

"I am?"

"Yes."

"You mean I won't die?"

"That's right. You're going to live."

LATER PAUL OBSERVED, "You smiled and the smile got bigger and bigger. You knew exactly what I was talking about. You were happy that you were going to live."

EVEN THOUGH Paul is on the hospital staff, it is unusual for a psychiatrist to be in the recovery room giving me the results of the operation before anyone else. Paul reads Simpson's chart entry and considers it "clear and conclusive." However, neither Simpson nor Aaron is going to tell me the results of the surgery until my spleen and sample lymph nodes are thoroughly examined by pathologists and a comprehensive report has been returned. This caution is understandable given the original misdiagnosis. But it means that even though they know the good news, they will not tell me until the following week, after the lab checks and double checks.

Will I live? Despite being thoroughly drugged, I understand—in a visceral way that medication cannot dull—that I am waiting for the answer. Paul decides that I am entitled to know as soon as the answer is available. So he tells me.

The information means that the cancer experience has changed from primarily physical to primarily emotional. Technology has more than an 80 percent chance of obliterating the disease. With these odds, the primary question now becomes: Will I needlessly allow the cancer experience to handicap me?

By giving the news, Paul is securing my trust so that in the months ahead I'll be willing to follow his lead and concentrate on a new agenda—recovery rather than survival.

Paul is also there because he cares about me. Today he regards it as acceptable to let down his professional guard and tell me he cares. He does it by giving the most important gift one can give another, the authoritative information: You will live. Paul's news report stays with me during the painful, disorienting, drugged days ahead, serving as a talisman to ward off depression and despair.

The anesthetic is slowly wearing off. Consciousness reluctantly reappears. I see Laura looking down over me, worried and concerned. I say, "Have you eaten?" She says not. I turn to the lady standing next to her. The woman looks familiar. I say to the lady, "Tell her to get something to eat." I awake again and the lady is still there. My mind takes a while to recognize who she is. She is my mother. I remember asking her to wait two days before visiting me. "What are you doing here?" I say. At that instant, the Rev. Mark Anderson, an Episcopal priest at St. Ann's Church, enters my field of vision. He is Robert's idea of a greeting card, and I smile at the notion. I watch Mother looking at his clerical collar, becoming disoriented and angry. Is she angry at me because I know a priest, or at Robert for converting?

My mind feels like the bank of a river with memories and thoughts streaming by at their own rate, sometimes too fast, sometimes too slow. I decide to stop thinking. I ask, "Did Laura get her sandwich?" and then fall asleep.

11

AFTER THE OPERATION, the fourth awakening is like no other. Returning to sleep is not possible. Staying awake is not bearable. There is just PAIN. Nothing matters but the pain. Its intensity is overwhelming. I scream. "The pain! The pain! It hurts! I want something for the pain!"

A nurse runs into the room and starts yelling at me. My ability to focus has not fully returned. The nurse has the jerky movements of a character in a silent movie. My sense of hearing doesn't seem to be working properly. I can tell that the nurse is yelling because her mouth is open so wide. She says (and I gather she's repeated the information several times before I understand), "You are full of morphine. You can't have any more medication. You don't need it." I say, "But I'm in pain!" I feel unable to control the volume of my voice. The nurse goes into a long explanation about pain, ending with, "You can't be in pain *yet*. You can't have more medication *yet*."

I had not anticipated *this*. There is a cut in my belly from the chest to below the belly button, and both under my skin and through it I feel a burning pain that gets hotter and more intense as the medication wears off. The pain is overwhelming. It creates waves of fear and incredulity in me. Before, pain had been instantaneous—a needle jabbing in my toes or under my arm. Pain lasted only until the anesthetic worked. Or, pain lasted a short period of time—long enough for Aaron to remove my bone marrow. Or, pain could be wiped out by medication, like after the arm operation. Now I have graduated to a new and higher order of pain.

Right then, at the moment of my fourth waking, Laura intervenes. She tells the nurse, "Stop telling him he doesn't hurt and find a doctor." The doctor decides I am entitled to more medication. After a short interminable wait the medication is inside me; the pain lessens.

I feel love for Laura. Laura is on my side. Laura loves me and doesn't want me in pain. Love, I decide, means less pain.

Of course the pain doesn't go away. It simply becomes less violent before becoming more violent. I am on a three-hour injection cycle. I can get medication only after waiting three hours and only if I ask for it.

I buzz repeatedly, asking the time, trying to make sure that I don't miss the injection and that the injection isn't late. Every time Simpson comes by to ask how I am doing, I ask for stronger pain medication, more frequently. He says the medication is as strong as it comes. "What's it called? Are you sure there isn't anything stronger? Can't you double the dosage or triple it?"

There was nothing on the release form I signed saying "We are not responsible for unbearable pain." I become preoccupied with pain. Death, I always assumed, would be quick and painless, but even if death were long and debilitating, it couldn't possibly hurt as much as this. Now that I know I will live, I regret ever deciding to save my life.

I am in pain even when I am asleep. I spend considerable time praying to God for relief of pain. Since I don't believe that God answers prayers, the prayers are a form of panic. I keep asking myself: What is pain? Why does it hurt? Why do I have to hurt so much? During the eleven days I am in the hospital, the pain doesn't stop.

I am on drugs the entire time. The drugs frequently make me feel incoherent. Sometimes they'll be strong enough so that the world is a blur. Time, events, and visitors themselves seem like characters in a disturbing dream. Too often, however, I feel that I am all too coherent. I don't want to be aware. I don't want to be conscious. I don't want to see anyone or do anything. I just want to be without pain.

I find that I can be in pain and uncomfortable at the same time. You know the old maxim about curing a toothache by cutting off your leg. Well it doesn't work. At least it doesn't work for long. While still incredulous about the intensity of the pain, I begin to notice the condition of my body.

Many of my visitors are frightened to see me all hooked up, unable to move, and looking like hell. No one is more frightened than I am. Two days earlier I considered riding a bicycle to the hospital. Now I am unable to walk. There is a tube up my nose, a tube in each arm, and a tube draining stuff out of my wound.

They had certainly explained the procedure to me. I guess they assumed I'd know about IV (intravenous) tubes and drainage pumps. And I assumed there would be a lot of stitches and a large bandage, that it would hurt for a day or two and I'd spend most of the time in bed before the wound healed. Well, that's not the way it works. Abdominal surgery is *major* surgery. It may be routine, but it is routine *major* surgery.

LAURA, who had gone to nursing school, later said she too was unprepared for the dramatic change in my appearance. "I have seen a lot of people coming out of surgery, so I thought I knew what to expect. But seeing all the tubes stuck in you was shocking. It made you look so vulnerable. It was scary. I thought the nurse was a bitch because she kept telling you that you weren't in any pain, that you had just had a pain-killer in the recovery room, and that you didn't need anything."

Of the days that followed, she said, "You were pretty dopey a lot of the time. You weren't responsive to people's conversations. I mean, often people would have conversations around you and it was like you weren't there.

"You looked pretty fragile. I was afraid. You were pale and thin and really weak. Your mother kept nagging at you, and it pissed me off that they were so nasty to you about pain-killers." She laughed. "I said to myself, 'This sucks. I was looking for a big, strong man.' "

BECAUSE of baby-sitter problems, Laura often brings the children over to the hospital, where they have long waits in the lobby. Children are not allowed to visit patients in their rooms. One evening, when I'm feeling well enough, Laura pushes me in a wheelchair. I glide into the lobby guiding the wheeled IV rack with my hand. I know I look terrible. I haven't shaved in days. I've lost weight. I am covered with bandages. I am pale.

The children look at me and they are frightened. I watch them watch me, imagining their words, *So this is what death looks like.*

KAREN REMEMBERED my disease as a series of long hospital waits. "I was waiting until Mommy came down because we weren't allowed to go up there," she said. "It was boring. There was nothing to do. She was up there a long time. I was mad that she was up there for so many hours."

Luke remembered: "Mom was awful mad at you because of the way you acted in the hospital. She was depressed. She thought you were acting badly, that you were expecting her to wait on you and that you kept complaining to her about the way the hospital was treating you. You complained about the food and how they wouldn't let you walk around. She said it hurt and they wouldn't give you anything for the pain and that you kept whining about the pain. Whenever she came back, she was mad. When I asked her why she was mad, she'd say, 'Joel's being an asshole.' " Luke paused and then, trying to take back what he'd just said, went on, "I don't want you to think that she didn't understand and feel sad about your disease and everything. I mean, maybe she didn't say that you were being an asshole. Maybe she said, 'I think he's being unreasonable.' "

My mother remembered: "I looked down at the bed that held this person who was my son. I couldn't believe what I saw—this son to whom I had given life and to whom I had given all that I could give anyone in the form of love. It was upsetting to see your weakened condition and all the bottles and tubes connected to you and to see the writhing and the venom and the anger spewing forth. You were drugged and groggy and screaming for pain-killers. You acknowledged my presence and screamed for pain-killers. I couldn't believe that this was my son and that this was happening. It had to have been a stranger, someone else."

I MEASURE THE DAYS by progress made recovering from the operation. Each day passes with agonizing slowness. First, the IV in my left arm is removed. That makes it possible to get out of bed, stand, and attempt to urinate into a bedpan. Standing and trying to urinate is ghastly. There are still too many tubes. Either I get tangled up or, worse yet, I pull at a tube. Meanwhile, I have to hold my abdomen—covered by an enormous bloody bandage with attached drainage tube and sack. The pain is staggering. On Thursday night, drugged and confused, I ask Laura to help me. She has her arm around me, helping to steady me as I am swaying. Standing with my penis dangling out, I say to Laura, "Please, piss for me."

"I can't," she says, frustrated that she is unable to help. "I don't know what to do." My bladder still full, I painfully return to bed.

All the next day, nurses and assorted medical students try to coax me to urinate. Sometimes I am lucid enough to feel embarrassed. I am often frustrated by the failure. No matter how hard I try, either nothing comes out or, worse, a little bit and it stops. A physician explains, "We'll have to catheterize you if you don't cooperate. We don't like to do that because of the risk of bladder infection. Also it helps your recovery from surgery if you move around."

By Friday night, I am getting panicky. My bladder is so full, I feel as if I'm about to explode. When I'm not thinking about the pain from the operation, I'm thinking of the pain from not urinating. On Saturday morning I am catheterized. I am feeling very uneasy as the medical student sticks a tube into my penis. I tell him to do it slowly. I tell him to be gentle. Then, *whoosh*—fifteen hundred cc's enters the sack at the end of the tube.

Meanwhile, someone takes the tube out of my nose. I am permitted to suck on chips of ice and to have small sips of water. A physical therapist comes by with a toy. It is a plastic device with three plastic balls inside. There is a mouthpiece attached, and by blowing air into the toy I raise the balls to the top. A feeble three-pack-a-day smoker can blow enough air to make the balls rise. I can't. My lungs are reluctant to hold air—it hurts to take deep breaths. The therapist tells me to cough from my diaphragm. I do. Once. But my diaphragm is where the incision is. The pain from coughing is spectacular. No, I won't cough again. No, I won't play with the blow bottle anymore. The therapist warns that unless I do what she says, my lungs will become filled with liquid. I do not listen to the horrors that will follow. I stop listening and tell her to go away.

By Sunday, my bandages are no longer drenched in blood. They need to be changed less frequently. That is good news, because changing the bandages hurts and the process frightens me. I find that I am frightened whenever anyone touches me. I begin to associate physical contact with pain and discomfort.

At some point, Simpson explains that abdominal surgery affects the necessity for a bowel movement. My wounds have to heal for three or four days before I'll feel "the urge to evacuate." On Monday, Memorial Day, they begin giving me a series of enemas. My body has to learn again about bowel movements. It is humiliating.

On Monday, I am put on a clear liquid diet. A note in my

chart orders the nurses to "encourage ambulation," which means they push me out of bed and into the blue fake-leather armchair by the side of the bed. Then they walk me around the hallway until I've had too much. Later that afternoon, Laura wheels me out onto the sixth-floor balcony.

I can't believe what I see. There is blue sky; a view of the Watergate complex, the Potomac River, and lots of trees. It is a beautiful surprise that anything exists—anything, that is, outside the drab room and corridor.

Tuesday is a big day. My mother goes back to Florida. I am given food to eat. The sutures are removed from my feet, where they were slit open for the lymphangiogram. The drainage tube is removed from my wound. I am disconnected from the catheter and the IV. Free at last!

Sometime that day Aaron comes by and explains the results of the operation. "The pathologist found no presence of Hodgkin's disease in your spleen and in the other samples Dr. Simpson took. That is good news." Aaron continues, "First, you'll be given radiation treatment. When that is over, I'll evaluate your progress and decide whether you also need chemotherapy. You don't have to see me again until the radiation treatment is over. I've set up an appointment for you to see the radiologist tomorrow. When you get out of the hospital, I want you to see Dr. Simpson in his office. He'll examine your wound and see that everything is all right."

That evening I begin to cry. My roommate, a Mr. Collier, asks whether I am all right. I say, "I'm fine. I just want to cry." He calls for a nurse. She wants to know what is wrong. "Nothing is wrong. I just want to cry." She wants to know what she can do to help. "You can leave me alone." She calls the resident.

The resident says, "Why are you crying?"

"I just want to cry."

She tells me to stop. "You are upsetting the other patients."

I tell her to get lost. Later, when I finish with the tears, I ring and ask to speak to the resident. Angry that anyone would dare ask me to stop crying, I yell, "You're what's wrong with doctors. You have no feelings." It feels good to shout at someone. Feeling good is a surprise.

On Wednesday, I am wheeled down to the basement to see Dr. Daniel Grey, chief of G.W.'s Division of Radiation Oncology. He briefly explains about radiation, saying that it takes place on an out-patient basis. He tells me not to procreate children while undergoing treatment. He asks his secretary to give me an appointment card.

On Thursday, the sutures are removed from my abdominal wound. I am given a pass to leave the building for a few hours. Slowly I walk the three blocks to group. On Friday I develop a urinary infection (because of the catheter). On Saturday, I am discharged from the hospital with a prescription for ampicillin for infection and a prescription for Percodan for pain. Simpson swears that Percodan is the strongest oral pain medication available.

I never wanted to leave a place as badly as I want to leave that hospital. Leaving is pure happiness. And, I am with Laura.

12

Y EARS LATER, after the radiation treatment was over, after my hair had grown back and my health seemed assured, Mother and I had a pleasant dinner alone together. I said to her, "You know you're really pleasant company." She said, "You say that as if you were surprised." I was. I had not realized that my mother was a pleasant and likable woman. Certainly not when I was still in the hospital.

DESPITE my clear insistence that Mother wait a day or two for me to recover from the operation, she is right there on the spot as soon as I awake from the anesthesia and begin screaming in pain. When I realize who she is, I am very angry. I had insisted, but there she is anyway.

Mother says, "I arrived at the hospital bright and early, with reading material and my *Siddur* [prayer book]. I was seated and ready to wait around the clock."

Mother has established a constant vigil by my bedside. I am not appreciative. I want to be alone. Since I have to be in pain, I prefer to do it without having a constant censorious audience. During the days that follow my operation, Mother arrives first thing in the morning and stays all day long. Frequently, she goes without food because she wants to be by my bedside. Often, she has to be coaxed and taken out by my other visitors to have a meal. Because Mother is continuously there, we fight incessantly. The fights are raw and ugly. My patience is nonexistent. For the first time since I was an infant, I am physically unable to move and take care of myself. Being forced to relive the powerlessness and helplessness of childhood is bad enough. Being required to do so in my mother's presence seems like a surrealist film director's idea of a bad joke. I feel humiliated by my immobility, and I feel angry.

I react to Mother's constant barrage of help, suggestions, and criticism with blanket negativity. I do not see her as someone who loves me and is concerned for my welfare. Instead I see her as someone who wants to interfere with my life and force me to do things I don't want to do. Some of her suggestions for my care may be valuable, but I am so overwhelmed by Mother's intensity that I am unable to appreciate the positive aspects of her concern.

Rationally, my insistence that Mother wait a few days was probably not realistic. From her perspective, how could she stay away from her only son when he was undergoing major surgery for a possibly fatal illness? I wasn't, however, feeling either rational or realistic. Indeed, I hadn't even wanted to tell Mother about my cancer and did so only after a series of verbal battles with Paul, in which I finally backed down. I justified telling Mother on the grounds that my psychiatrist strongly recommended it, and if I didn't want to follow his recommendations, why was I going to him?

In February, when I told Mother I planned to marry Laura, she said, "I'd prefer you dead." Now that it was May and there appeared some chance she might get her wish, I didn't want to make her feel guilty. I no longer needed her approval of my relationship with Laura. What I wanted from her was to let go, to accept my right to lead my own life and make my own mistakes. My cancer, I feared, presented an open invitation to meddle. I resented the idea of telling Mother about something of major importance in my life. Having told her, I hoped she would restrain her instincts and respect my wishes.

After a few days of watching me request Meperdine injections every three hours, Mother has a discussion with one of the nurses. They decide that I am at risk of becoming a dope addict. Mother says, "We think you should deal with pain without medication." The idea of being without drugs panics me. The pain is bad enough with the medication; having the medication stopped and having Mother be the one to stop it seems the worst imaginable nightmare. I demand (a word too mild for my near-hysteria) that my doctors—one by one as they arrive—order the do-gooder nurse to stop interfering with my medication. I also demand that the nursing staff be ordered to stop discussing my medical condition with my mother. "All reports on me should be channeled through Laura." The nurse gets the message. My mother doesn't.

Mother's setback about the medication adds intensity to her conclusion that my doctors do not know what they are doing but that she does. Her failure at reaching them only intensifies her efforts. Aaron, Simpson, and their colleagues react either by giving curt responses to her demands for information or by avoiding her. She then tries to reach Paul to convince him that she is the only one interested in my welfare and that he should tell me to listen to my mother. After their second conversation, Paul makes himself unavailable to her. Mother takes out this series of rebuffs on me, complaining that my physicians are hostile and incompetent. When I say, "But Mother, they're only following instructions," she resumes arguing with me.

Mother's attitude is clear and persistent. She believes that I am incapable of taking care of myself or knowing my own mind. So she decides that she will take over. She wants me to go back to Florida with her.

"I can take care of you down there. You know we have plenty of fine physicians down there. You can have your radiation therapy and your chemotherapy in Florida, and there's plenty of room for you to stay." She begins describing the privacy I can enjoy living in her new apartment. She is already moving around the furniture.

Mother gives the impression that she will allow nothing to interfere with her dramatic debut as the Martyred Parent. Whether I want it or not, she is going to nurse me through the long and agonizing months ahead until I die with dignity. Of course, she doesn't actually say that I am going to die. Instead she gives me so many intense reassurances that their phoniness becomes apparent. She will nurse me as she nursed her father, who died when he was a young man. Both at my bedside and alone with Laura, Mother talks about my grandfather (which she rarely does). It is a closely held family secret that my grandfather was not Jewish. "He died with dignity," she tells me. That fact that I am neither going to die nor be dignified does not seem to have reached her. She is there to force dignity upon me.

WHAT I DIDN'T REALIZE at the time was that because Laura didn't trust Aaron and because an undercurrent of hostility existed between them, the good news of my operation results got garbled. After all, Laura was the spokesman for my condition and I had instructed the doctors not to brief Mother while I was in the hospital. So, Laura, Mother, relatives and friends were unclear about my chances of living. I knew what my chances were, but I was in no condition to give a lucid explanation.

WHEN LAURA VISITS ME, Mother tries to elicit her support in convincing me to go to Florida for treatment. When Laura isn't present, Mother vilifies Laura, detailing all the faults she can find, from Laura's housekeeping to the way her children dress.

She tells me to end my relationship with Laura. She says that Laura represents everything wrong with my life and my values. She recites a long catalog of why the relationship with Laura is "wrong."

INTERMARRIAGE and sickness—and the connections she made between them—evoked in Mother overwhelming emotion. Mother was the daughter of a sixteen-year-old Jewish girl who ran off with a saxophone player. Yes, he really was a saxophone player. He was also Italian, and my grandmother's parents—in keeping with Jewish tradition—mourned her as dead when she married a gentile. When Mother was born, the marriage had already begun to sour and my guilty grandmother regarded her daughter's birth as proof of her guilt. Shortly thereafter, my grandfather became sick with what later was diagnosed as Parkinson's disease. That he was in fact sick was not clear for years. His behavior, however, appeared to be dangerously irrational, and Grandmother fled to her Jewish parents. There she and Mother were taken in, but made to feel the extent of their "shame." Mother was teased by her cousins for being "half Jewish" and a "*shiksa*," and she reacted by excelling in Hebrew studies and becoming a Hebrew school teacher, by making herself unmistakably Jewish.

Meanwhile my grandfather was placed in an understaffed public hospital where he slowly died. Mother sneaked out to visit and nurse her father, afraid to tell her mother and Jewish relatives what she was doing. Later, when I was born, I was named for my Italian grandfather without my father ever realizing it. Mother translated *Salvatore* into Hebrew and came up with *Joel Ezra*. According to a complicated logic, which I never understood, I was supposed to step into my grandfather's role, only I was supposed to be so Jewish and so successful that it would rid Mother of the shame of having a gentile father. Therefore I was somehow betraying my gentile grandfather, my heritage, and my mother by becoming involved with a gentile. On top of that, my getting sick—as my grandfather had—made Mother recall a flood of sad memories.

Clearly, Mother was frightened. She acted strong and domineering because that was her way of dealing with fear. Today I realize that Mother's fear had made her feel weak and vulnerable—that the degree of intensity with which she tried to control me was a measure of the depth of her fear. But at the time I wasn't feeling sensitive to her needs. I was caught up in my own.

MY POWERLESSNESS makes me feel strongly tempted to give in to Mother, to have her take me away from the misery of the hospital bed to a clean and comfortable apartment in Florida where she will attentively take care of me. But I know in some visceral way that if I give in I'll become an emotional cripple—that giving in will retard my ability to return to a normal adult life. The disease gives me the choice: either I can use it as an excuse to avoid responsibility or I can accept the disease as yet another inconvenience. Because Mother will be content with nothing but full capitulation to her wishes, I feel that the only position I can take is say no to everything she suggests. The more I say no, the more rigid she becomes. Soon our arguments leave the subject of disease and care. We have said all there is to say. So we begin to argue about peripheral issues. We argue about Robert, whose parents were friends of Mother's. We argue about Laura's children. We argue about God. We rehash my marriage. We rehash her marriages. All the old, tired, forgotten issues that families keep locked up for decades are brought out again. We hurl them at each other simply to hurt each other.

This unattractive spectacle does not take place in private. Mother has called in her relatives, and I begin to feel myself the object of a family pilgrimage. Relatives I haven't seen in years are unexpectedly at my bedside. Waking from a drugged sleep I see Cousin Phyllis, whom I don't recognize at first. Theresa and Alvin, who never leave Manhattan, suddenly get on a plane and shuttle down. Other relatives, Mother assures me, are on stand-by, waiting to arrive on my say-so. "No," I say. "I don't think it is necessary for Uncle Jack to come down, as kind as it is of him to offer."

Also visiting me is Laura's family—her mother, sister, sister's lover, brother Matthew, brother Lionel. Andy and Patric and Robert come. Robert sends his friends. My father sends his stepdaughter Susan. The members of my group are there.

The visitors frequently serve as a backdrop for my battles with Mother. Mother tries to get the visitors to agree that I am treating her badly. I in turn complain about Mother. At one point Andy says to me, "Is there anything I can do?" Before I can answer he says, "Yes, I can get your mother out of the room and take her for a drive."

Mother's constant battling is difficult for her. She feels alone and needy of someone else. The visitors are temporaries. The only other person who is constantly there is Laura. So Mother turns to Laura for comfort and support. Outside the hospital is neutral territory. Laura and Mother go out to suppers together and have long talks.

When Mother asked Laura to make hotel reservations, she made Laura promise not to tell me that she was coming up earlier than I wanted. Mother feels that because she is a partner with Laura in their shared secret, it has brought them closer together.

Mother says, "She is kind enough to find me suitable accommodations at the hotel. Our relationship is a good one person to person. She is most hospitable."

One night, at Laura's house, Mother refuses to drink any wine. Instead, she complains about me, how hard life is, and how difficult her childhood was. She tries to explain to Laura why she is so opposed to intermarriage. "You see," she says, revealing the dark secret, "my father was a gentile." Laura jumps up and laughs. "That's rich. That's really rich. That's the funniest thing I've ever heard. Your father was a gentile. That explains everything." Then Mother grabs the wine bottle saying, "Give me some of that."

They become, in their own way, buddies.

On Tuesday, June 1, when I am still in the hospital, Mother finally goes back home. It is a bitter leave-taking. She gives me an open invitation to nursing care in Florida, knowing that I will never accept. She is angry. She says, "You've become a stranger to me."

She says, "I know that you will get well. When you are physically well then maybe your emotions will be healthier. The sickest part of you is not the Hodgkin's disease, which invaded a part of your body. One day everything will change. Laura will understand. You will understand. And I hope I will survive the pain of the things I have endured to see that day."

$$\boxed{13}$$

O<small>N THE FIRST SATURDAY</small> in June, Laura pulls her green Volkswagen bug up to the hospital's Twenty-second Street entrance, where I am waiting in a wheelchair. The wheelchair is unnecessary, but the hospital insists. In character to the end, I resent the insistence. The nurse who pushes the wheelchair helps Laura load the car with flowers, books, assorted gifts, and personal belongings.

I thumb through the seven-page computer printout of the bill, which I was required to sign before being released. The doctors' bills will come later.

The total is $3,550.52 for room and board for eleven days and nights. The bill frightens me. I worry about whether my insurance really does exist. If so, will it cover the bill? I decide against worrying and stuff the bill packet somewhere in the car.

I believe the worst is over. I know I am going to survive

the disease, and I feel well enough to be happy about it. I think that all I have to do is recover from the operation, which I am doing nicely. Slowly, my energy is returning. I am impatient.

I feel intense liberation as we drive away. I rip at the plastic bracelet. When it refuses to come off instantly, I gnaw at it with my teeth. The day is beautiful. The drive is beautiful. The trees in Rock Creek Park are beautiful.

As I cautiously lift myself out of the car and slowly walk upstairs to Laura's bedroom, I feel that I have survived the major battle of a war. When I get better, I promise myself, I'll finish my agriculture book. I'll finish my article assignments. I'll do my consulting work. I'll find a good job. I'll marry Laura. I'll be a father to her children.

I make intricate plans for the future, cheerfully thinking about what I want to do and how I am going to enjoy life.

Life suddenly seems like a brand new gift. I have been given a second chance. Ahead seems hope and opportunity. Soon, the pain of the operation will be gone. Soon I will stop thinking about me, me, me and include Laura in my life, giving to Laura, returning to her the love she gives to me.

We make love in her king-size bed. The sex is awkward and slow. It is painful for me to move. I keep worrying, holding my belly, afraid that my newly healed scars will give in to gravity and my insides will burst. Such concerns interfere. Laura suggests, "Maybe we should wait until you feel better." No. I won't wait. I am obsessed with the idea of having sex, with proving to myself that sex is possible and that I can satisfy her.

We both become very frustrated. Our movements aren't coordinated. It is mechanical in the worst possible way. Our timing is off and our tempers become frayed. But I refuse to stop. Eventually, pleasure overcomes all obstacles. We both marvel at how wonderful pleasure is.

Gingerly, I inspect myself to make sure that I am undamaged. Satisfied, I inspect Laura and admire her. Again, I feel glad to be alive. I tell myself, *Remember life is joy and pleasure and love.* I tell myself, *Do not forget.* I promise myself that I will always appreciate life.

On Sunday afternoon, Laura looks at my belly. She says, "Let me look at that again. Your wound looks red. It looks angry."

"It's nothing."

"It is puffy and probably infected."

"It will keep until Tuesday when I have an appointment with Simpson."

"It won't keep. You should call your doctor."

We argue. I sulk. I finally give in. I agree to call, but who is my doctor? I finally decide to call Aaron.

The answering service takes the message. One of Aaron's associates returns the call. I say, "It's probably nothing, but my lady friend insists that the wound looks red." I hand the phone to Laura. She describes the wound.

The doctor says, "I want you to go the hospital right away. Can your friend drive you to the emergency room?" I don't want to go back to the hospital.

"Is it necessary? Can't I wait until Tuesday?"

Laura drives me to the hospital.

The emergency room is dismal, but not as dismal as I expected. There are the usual form-filling questions—date of birth, insurance number, occupation. The wait is long, but not as long as I feared. Only after the wait do things seem worse than imagined.

The physician explains that I have a wound infection. She says, "I'm going to open up the incision and clean out the area."

I stall. I do not want to be touched. I do not want my belly slit open again. I do not want the pain she is going to inflict. I do not want a strange doctor working on me. "Can't I wait until tomorrow and see my regular doctor?"

She says, "Your wife can leave the room now."

"She's not my wife; I want her to stay." I am afraid of being left alone. I squeeze Laura's hand as the doctor slits open the wound where it is red. She drains out five cc's of pus.

"What they did," Laura says later, "was revolting. They lanced it. I thought I was going to faint. I got real sick and hot."

Afterward the doctor puts on a large bandage and tells me to make an appointment with my surgeon. When I go back to Laura's my own odor nauseates me. I don't want to be around anyone smelling like that, with a large stinking bandage. I want to be alone, to hide until I get better. I decide to go back to my apartment. I ask Laura to drive me there on Monday morning.

THAT WAS a mistake.

What I should have done was stay at Laura's house. I should have trusted Laura. I should have let myself believe the truth, that no matter how disgusted I was with my own body and no matter how humiliated I felt by the infection, Laura loved me and would care for me.

The wound infection was just one indication that the worst was not over. I still had difficulty moving around. I was going to have difficulty shopping for myself, cooking for myself, getting the medical supplies I needed. Soon the infection and the difficulties would become worse. Soon the radiation would start and my energy would disappear.

By giving in to the impulse for familiar surroundings and aloneness, I was making it extremely difficult for Laura to care for me. It took her nearly an hour to drive from her house on the Maryland line to my apartment on Capitol Hill; I did not own a car, and there was no quick, reliable public transportation. Since Laura had children to care for and cats to feed, she would often drive downtown to work, back up to her house, across town to my apartment, and then back home.

Then there was the real and symbolic importance of Laura's house. Earlier that year, on one particularly stupid and egocentric evening, I insisted on spending the night at her house. She fought my insistence, but not hard enough. The children told Daddy. It became a critical point in the negotiations. Jim insisted on requiring in the settlement (which gave Laura the right to live in her house) Laura's written agreement that she not "live with a man." It was probably not legal, nor enforceable.

However, that summer was the first time since the divorce that Jim had full-time custody of the children. Laura feared that if we lived together, Jim would not return the children and he would order the sale of the house. My cancer effectively wiped out that problem. The children had told Jim about my cancer. He told them how sorry he was and frequently asked about my health. Certainly Jim wasn't going to be vindictive to his former wife's "dying" boyfriend. That wasn't in Jim's nature, and Laura knew it. So I could have stayed in the house. Laura could have taken care of me. I could have played with the children in the evenings until summer vacation and their time with Jim. After the children had gone to Jim's, Laura's concern for the house and the possible risk of leaving made her fearful of moving into my small apartment. By leaving Laura's house, I was giving up a rare opportunity to live with Laura and see whether it could work out.

ON MONDAY MORNING, Laura drives me to my apartment. Her car is filled with the gifts, flowers, and possessions I brought to her house from the hospital. After helping unload, she is impatient to leave. She has to go to work. Sitting alone in the apartment, I feel panicked and deserted.

I have to call Simpson about the infection. There is also work I want to do, am impatient to do. I have to call back the sugar lawyer in New York. I have to write the article on the agriculture department for *The Washingtonian*. I have to answer the angry letters about the Cesar Chavez article.

THE ARTICLE, entitled "Can Chavez Cope With Success?", was unflattering. When I went to California to research agricultural labor, I wanted to like him. I found that Chavez was neglecting the day-to-day problems of his union membership, masking them with heavy doses of rhetoric. There was also his public image as a saintly pacifist, contrasted with the intimidation I had felt interviewing Chavez in a room where his guard dog waited, a dog he had personally trained to attack on command. *The New Republic* was flooded with dozens of irate letters, which Laura brought me in the hospital. Nuns especially wanted to know how I could criticize such a holy man. In the hospital, I sometimes felt like one of those characters who messed with Philadelphia's Father Divine. God will get you for this.

THE MORNING hasn't even begun, and already I am tired. My body is telling me to rest, but I am not going to pay attention. I sit waiting for the energy to return and waiting for myself to develop a plan on how to spend the day. I stare at the stuffed animal Laura gave me as a present in the hospital. It is a beautiful monkey, with arms outstretched as if to embrace someone. The monkey makes me feel sad, yet somehow it comforts me. I believe the monkey understands me, and Laura knows that. Looking at the monkey makes me feel sentimental about Laura. Will I ever feel as close to her as I do to this stuffed animal?

I call Simpson's office and am given an appointment for that morning. He tells me not to worry. He says that I should take baths, that I should soak and then wash out the area that is still draining pus. Despite the enormous emergency-room bandages, the site of the infection, when I get a good look at the wound, is not very big. I am hopeful that the problem will clear up shortly. At the pharmacy, I stock up on squares of surgical gauze and tape.

I spend Monday and Tuesday running around town. The New York lawyer asks me to do some research. So I go to the Securities and Exchange Commission, to the agriculture department, and to the Library of Congress. I am eager to test out my body. I walk when I can take the bus. I run when I can walk. I am too impatient to take elevators, so I climb stairs. By Tuesday, I am exhausted. I have always been impatient, always on the run. This time, however, I have been hospitalized for eleven days and do not consider that my body needs to recover. And it works like a vicious circle. When I tire, I become frightened, so I push myself even harder.

On Tuesday night I go over to Robert's house for supper. He lives in Rosslyn—across the street from the Iwo Jima Monument—in a two-bedroom apartment, which he painted chocolate brown and filled with fashionable furniture. He shares the place with his lover Ron and with Allen, who pays the rent and whom I like.

Ron and I do not get along. He doesn't like straight people. He doesn't treat Robert well. He knows Robert and I are confidants, and he resents our frequent reminiscenses about our childhood. He is not at all pleased that Robert has invited a cancer patient to dinner and makes no attempt to hide his displeasure.

Robert is worrying about pleasing Ron and being pleasant to me at the same time. Although the evening is noticeably awkward, the awkwardness goes unmentioned. Robert, Allen, and I are louder than we need be. Allen, who spent many hours at the hospital visiting me as Robert's proxy, tells amusing stories about my mother and about how silly I looked with tubes stuck in me. Before dessert, I excuse myself to go to the bathroom.

While adjusting the bandage, pus begins oozing from my belly along much of the wound line and even to the side of it. I am terrified. I have never seen so much pus before. My own body is disgusting and I nearly vomit. I call out to Robert, who comes to the bathroom door. I tell him that I'll be in the bathroom for a while and to have dessert without me.

I take a bath, washing out the infected area, terrified that my belly will simply burst apart. I am close to tears. I want to die. I want to do anything that will stop the feeling of horror and disgust at my own body. Gradually I calm down and return to the living room with a towel stuffed under my shirt.

I am panicked and exhausted. I tell Robert, Allen, and

Ron about the wound infection and the sudden inexplicable oozing. Ron excuses himself for the evening. Robert is mildly hysterical. In calming him down, I help calm myself down.

Robert says, "Why don't you sleep on the living-room couch? In the morning I'll drive you home." I agree. After converting the couch into a bed, Robert puts on the sheets, gives me the additional towels I requested, and then he and Allen say good-night. Using the kitchen telephone, I call Laura. I say, "I love you," wanting her to say she loves me. Covering myself with towels and then with a sheet, I am frightened. Sleep comes slowly.

Wednesday is a work day. I seize the only bathroom as soon as I awake. Allen pounds on the door. "I have to go to work." Robert knocks, slightly apologetic, letting me know his schedule and explaining that Ron also has to use the bathroom. I am in the bathtub, washing out the pus that has seeped out overnight. Slowly, grudgingly, I get dressed, cover my belly with a towel, and leave the bathroom.

As Robert drives me back to my apartment, I know that my behavior has put distance between us. Robert overcame considerable fear in visiting me in the hospital. Now that I am out and am seeking his help, he feels at once angry and guilty. I know that in the immediate future Robert will see as little of me as he possibly can.

ROBERT LATER TOLD ME, "That time I had you over for dinner was a disaster. I was torn between comforting you and avoiding Ron's resentment. Ron couldn't handle it, and besides, you were just awful. You were impossible to deal with. You were very short-tempered and you were very demanding.

"There was a conflict between Ron and me. He made his

resentment known. He said if I wanted to be with you, I should be with you on your own territory, and he didn't want to deal with it. Although I felt emotionally dependent on him, I wanted to be with you. But, on the other hand, I couldn't be with you to the point of provoking his hostility.

"Laura made my job easier. She was your primary relationship. She was very attentive. She was there all the time. It made it easier for me to know that she was taking care of you. After all, I had my own preoccupations. A lot of real craziness was going on with me, my vocation, and Ron." He laughed. "I mean, I was emotionally dependent on a homosexual lover and, at the same time, I was entering a celibate religious order. There was an inherent conflict there. Yet, somehow I managed to obscure that in brocade and incense."

ON WEDNESDAY MORNING, feeling close to hysteria, I go to a hastily requested appointment with Simpson. Not only is the wound infected, but I am having an allergic reaction.

The problem probably began immediately after the operation, when Simpson sewed me up using two sets of sutures. The first set, deep below the skin line, literally held my abdomen closed. The second set was at the surface. In the hospital, after the wound on the surface had healed, those sutures were removed. There remain the set of permanent sutures deep inside. Most surgery patients never realize that sutures remain inside long after the wounds have healed. I, however, am allergic to the sutures. Some are bubbling to the surface, where they contribute to the wound infection and have to be pulled out.

Simpson grabs a string with his tweezer—a string that is partially sticking out, right at my belly button. Last night I tugged at it, not realizing that it was a suture—afraid that if I pulled too hard, I'd unravel.

Simpson puts scissors between the loop in the suture, snips, and pulls it out. He searches for additional sutures, cutting into my wound with his scalpel. After probing around and adjusting a lamp several times so he can see, he finds more.

This ad-hoc surgery hurts, and I scream. Impossible as it may seem, I feel more sensitive to pain now than before. "Veterans are always more squeamish," Simpson says. He tells me to take Percodan for the painful burning in my belly. "I want you to continue to take baths and to soak the wound for at least ten minutes each time, twice a day. It will probably heal. If you don't get better, I'll put you back on the operating table, where I can see properly and can do the job right. Then we can search for more sutures." He makes it sound like a treasure hunt.

I don't want another operation. I don't want to have an infected body. I want this whole disgusting problem to go away.

Slowly, over the next two weeks, the infection clears up. Even then, a small spot—just above my belly button—continues to ooze pus. The radiologists consider delaying treatment, but decide to go ahead. The spot finally disappears. However, on and off for months, it unexpectedly reappears, bringing pus and infection, causing me to feel humiliated and frustrated.

SOMETIMES, I felt that this was the worst part of the cancer experience. I was wrong. It was merely a nuisance—an unpleasant side effect to routine diagnostic procedure. The worst was still ahead.

14

RADIATION TREATMENT was the worst experience of my life.

AT 8:30 a.m., Thursday, June 17, I reluctantly return to George Washington University Hospital and take a large slow elevator down one floor to the basement. Lost again in the rubble of construction, I finally find the route—past the PHARMACY (room G332) PLANT OPERATIONS (G333), LINEN (G334), and the NURSES' LOCKERS (G335). Turning right, I enter the DIVISION OF RADIATION ONCOLOGY & BIOPHYSICS (G342).

At the reception desk, Violet, the departmental nurse, is ready for me. I called her several times, canceling appointments, but I can delay no longer. Violet is quick and efficient, and she can be abrasive in protecting the dignity of the department's doctors. Taking my chart out, she marches me over to the changing room, explaining how to put on the ugly green hospital gown. "You can keep on your underwear, socks, and shoes."

She leads me down the corridor, past a blackboard with my name and disease in chalk, and into the simulator room (G354). The sign on the door reads:

THIS ROOM IS LEAD SHIELDED AS FOLLOWS:

Location	*Lead*
Door & Frame	¼"
Threshold	¼"

Beaneath that is a bright yellow sign: CAUTION HIGH RADIATION AREA, and below that: RADIATION. THIS EQUIPMENT PRODUCES IONIZING RADIATION WHEN ENERGIZED. The signs are misleading. The room is a simulator. The real machine and the real need for warning is through the next door, where, next Tuesday, I am scheduled to receive my first dose of radiation.

According to the chart, Dr. Grey, radiologist, is now my physician. A radiologist, my dictionary told me, is a physician specializing in the use of radiant energy to diagnose and treat disease. Grey is chief of his department's twenty-five-person staff and one of four radiologists. He is my physician of record for radiology treatment because Aaron specifically referred me to him.

Two weeks ago, when I first met Grey, I was still a patient in the hospital. The interview was brief; he didn't tell me much, and I was heavily sedated with much-desired mind-numbing drugs.

Today, I assume that Grey and I will go to his office and talk. He enters the simulator room, briefly looks down at me from over the top of his reading glasses, says hello, and leaves.

I ask one of the technologists whether I'll be seeing him later. She says, "Do you have an appointment?"

"No."

"I'll ask Violet."

Violet comes in and says, "Do you have a problem?"

"No. I was just wondering whether I am going to see Dr. Grey when I'm done."

"Well, he's very busy today. You need to make an appointment if you want to see him. Of course, if you have a specific problem, we have doctors on staff. If you need to see one for any reason, let me know."

In the simulator room, I lie down on a long table beneath a nine-foot-high machine waiting for the technologists to begin. The technologists are all attractive women in their mid-twenties. They are busy and full of youthful energy. Lying on the cold hard table, onto which I have climbed with difficulty, I feel like an eighty-year-old man. The women tell me their names, but I don't really pay attention. I think of them as *those young people* and am grateful that they are pleasant and don't bother me too much.

A technologist tattoos a small dot at the base of my chest. My body is slid back and forth on the machine. Low-level X rays are taken. Measurements are checked and double checked. After an hour, I am free to go.

LATER THAT DAY, I go to group and complain.

When I was in the hospital and received a pass to attend group, I was applauded when I arrived. Jack said he was delighted that the operation came out so well. Paul called on the group members to express, one by one, how they felt about my operation and to describe their fears.

At the time, my friend Andy asked about the group's reaction to the cancer. He was amused. "Jesus, that must have been a show stopper. Here everyone was all set to complain about their mothers, and you come along and say, 'I have cancer.' That must have shut them up." Actually, it did. Paul used my cancer as a way of focusing the group's attention on problems other than their own. It was a way of saying that some problems are physical, require more than psychological treatment, and must be attended to immediately.

Now my situation has changed. I am being treated. I will probably live. Paul will no longer let me use cancer as a way of upstaging the problems of Frank, Doris, Sally, Lois, Mona, and the other members of the group.

I am still grateful to Paul for visiting me in the hospital and assuring me that I will live. I now have a reputation as one who faced significant danger and dealt with it well. Although I don't want to damage the group's respect for me, I want relief from my fear.

I complain. The infection terrifies me. The upcoming radiation scares me. "After the surgery, Aaron disappeared," I tell Paul. "I now consider you and not Aaron my primary physician. I've known you longer. I trust you. I know you'll be there when I need you."

"I'm not your primary physician," Paul says. "Aaron is. If you don't like the way you're being treated or if you need any additional information on your medical condition, you should talk to Aaron."

"Will you call Aaron for me? Will you tell him that I'm worried?"

Paul says he will.

Later that day, I start hiccuping uncontrollably. Terrified, I race over to Aaron's office without an appointment. I tell him about the infection. "Also, I'm afraid of the radiation. I don't understand what the radiologists are going to do to me."

Aaron trys to calm me down, telling me to breathe into a paper bag. The hiccuping subsides.

"I'll be glad to talk to you anytime you want," Aaron says. "Just ask the receptionist for an appointment. I'll have her try to fit you into my schedule for the same day you call. However, I can't clear up your wound infection. You should rely on Dr. Simpson for that. I'm not in charge of your radiation treatment. Dr. Grey is. You should talk to him about that." Aaron says that he doesn't need to see me until the first set of radiation treatments is over—more than a month from now.

AARON RECENTLY OBSERVED, "If I learned one thing from our relationship, it's that the role of being a primary physician is a serious one. When you are the primary physician, you must take control over every event. You cannot simply be the administrator of that person's health—shuffling papers, consulting, giving pathological opinions, putting them in order, and coming up with a paper-derived conclusion. A physician does his best work when he is personally involved in every aspect of his patient's management."

At the time, however, I didn't think Aaron was doing that. Instead I saw him as an administrator who had absented himself from my care. I could have changed that. I could have told him what I thought and why I was angry.

However, I was testing people to prove that they cared, trying to see how much of my complaining they could take. I feared that Aaron had given up responsibility for my health, that Simpson was unable to control the infection, that Grey didn't care about his radiation patients. I thought that Paul was saying that my cancer wasn't his problem. Laura, I felt, was on the other side of town when I needed her. I believed that my doctors, Laura, Robert, and my other friends had deserted me. Since everyone has abandoned me, I concluded, asking for help means asking for rejection. I was filled with self-pity.

BY TUESDAY, June 22, after days of measuring and positioning, I am ready for treatment. At 10:45 A.M., wearing a hospital gown, I enter room G356, labeled LINEAR ACCELERATOR. The room has an additional cautionary sign: PATIENTS WITH CARDIAC PACEMAKERS MUST INFORM THEIR PHYSICIANS BEFORE ENTERING THE TREATMENT ROOM. Trudie, the technologist, pulls out a stepping stool so I can climb onto the table.

The machine is a Clinac-4 Linear Accelerator made by the Varian Corporation. It is capable of bombarding my body with up to 4 million volts of radioactive power.

Its size is frightening. I am lying on a table about four and one-half feet from the floor. Trudie slides the table forward into the center of the machine. Eight feet wide and nine feet tall, the machine is in front, on top, and below me. It has a disklike device, attached to a motorized swivel. As I remain stationary in the center, the entire machine can be turned in a complete circle. When I lean back, I can see a clocklike device, numbered from zero to 360 degrees, telling the technologist whether the machine is exactly above me, exactly below me, or at another angle.

Trudie lines me up so I present a clear target. Above is a square opening from which the X-ray beam will come out.

Two thin wires evenly divide the square, indicating where the beam's exact center will be.

My first set of treatments involves bombarding my body from the top of my neck to the base of my chest (where the tattoo mark is) and again from behind—a body area called the "mantle field." Bombarding the lymph nodes in the neck and under the arms with high-energy X rays provides technical problems. The purpose of the radiation is to kill lymph nodes, that is, to kill enough of them so the cancerous ones are destroyed. However, how do you kill lymph nodes without, at the same time, destroying or damaging the esophagus, thyroid, and lungs? The answer: shield the areas you don't want to hit with leadlike blocks.

The blocks were constructed in a back room by a staff member who used my measurements in shaping them from molds, after pouring molten liquid from a machine that looks like a coffeepot. These molds had to match the X rays of my lungs. Then the blocks were mounted on two Plexiglas boards, one for my front and one for my back.

As I lie on the table, Trudie takes out the front set of blocks and slides it into the machine just below the square opening. Then she tapes a copper strip onto the Plexiglas. This serves as a partial shield, so that even though the neck is thinner than the torso, they both get equal doses. The Plexiglas, with its taped copper strips, seems such an amateur device compared to the sophisticated equipment all around me. It gives the queasy impression that the people running the machines don't know what they're doing.

Trudie lines up my body so it is exactly beneath the opening and the metal blocks are in the right place to protect my lungs and thyroid. She turns on a light, located inside the opening. It shows her the exact place the invisible radiation beam will hit. Her task is easier because on Monday I was marked with purple dye lines, turning both sides of my body into targets.

After making certain my body is in the right place and after telling me again not to move, Trudie literally runs out of the room. She locks the door. My neck is stretched all the way back, like that of a prisoner presenting himself for decapitation. After asking several questions, I was told that moving would put me off center and could cause the beam to burn an irreparable hole in my throat and other irreplaceable places. Thinking about possible disasters, I lie as still as possible, trying to concentrate on being still—an exercise that makes me restless.

Trudie is sitting at a console that has a television screen. She can use a remote control to turn the television camera pointed at my body and see whether I have moved. She switches on the intercom. "Are you all right?"

"Yes."

"Now hold still and I'll tell you when it's over." She turns a key, giving access to the machine's power source. She pushes the power switch. I hear a loud accelerating mechanical growl like the sound of an automobile in third gear when you push the accelerator to 60 mph and forget to shift to fourth.

Two yellow lights inside the room flash on, warning that if I want to avoid radiation I am too late. I am frightened by the machine, the blocks, the purple dye, the warning lights, and whatever this invisible beam is going to do to me. I am also frightened in general—frightened of things I cannot name. After a very long minute, the warning lights go off and the noise stops. Trudie reenters the room.

"That's it?" I ask, incredulous.

"That's it for that side. Now we have to do the other side."

"But I didn't feel anything."

"You're not supposed to feel anything."

"But it didn't hurt. I didn't feel any pain."

"I told you it wouldn't hurt."

Of course I didn't believe her. So far, virtually everything connected with the cancer experience has been painful. I think, *This isn't going to be bad.*

Trudie takes out the first set of blocks and inserts the second. She then helps turn me on the table so I am lying on my front, with arms to my sides and my chin tucked in. Again, my neck seems in a good position for an execution. As I stare down into the machine, I see a little window. Next to the window is a red sticker: CAUTION. LASER. DO NOT LOOK DIRECTLY INTO THE LASER AS IT MAY BE HARMFUL TO THE EYE. I look up, practically staring into the roof of my head as Trudie talks into the intercom and as I again hear the accelerating growl.

$$\boxed{15}$$

T HE FIRST WEEK is filled with the promise of things getting worse. "Oh, you don't have to worry about your hair falling out. That won't happen for weeks." To make matters worse, my physicians are uncertain how long treatment will take, and I worry that it will never end.

The schedule—subject to revision—calls for two sets of radiation treatment. The first is targeted between my neck and chest. The second will be at my abdomen. Each set will take about six weeks, give or take a few days (or weeks). The radiologists can't tell exactly because they don't know how sick I will get.

I am certain to lose weight, appetite, blood cells, and strength. Every Thursday I am weighed and a blood sample is taken. Every week the doctors decide whether I am strong enough to continue treatment. The dosimetrists have used computers to prescribe a total upper body dose of 3,963 rads.

That comes to 180 rads a day, administered Monday through Friday for about four weeks. However, if my body gets too sick from the daily dose, it might be necessary to stop for a day, a week, or longer until I am healthy enough to be resubjected to the sickness that continued treatment will cause.

If my entire body were bombarded with 180 rads, it would be three times greater than a fatal dose. However, the radiation is not fatal because it is directed to specific, relatively small areas of my body. The radiation—in the form of a high-energy X-ray beam—kills everything it hits. Specifically, it kills cells in designated portions of the lymphatic system. The X-ray beam cannot distinguish between "good" cells and "bad" cells. As a result, many healthy cells are killed—making the patient sick. The radiologists assume the result will be beneficial even though it makes the patient sick, because in the long run healthy cells will probably increase to a normal level and cancerous cells will probably have been obliterated. The nature and location of my disease provide high odds in favor of this assumption. There is, of course, no guarantee. I could be one of the statistically few—admittedly a very small number— who die or are permanently damaged by radiation treatment.

My fellow radiation patients may not be as lucky as I am. Their forms and locations of cancer may not prove accessible, partially or entirely, to the X-ray beam. For them, radiation may be a way of gaining time until the cancer returns. Or it may be an act of desperation—something for physicians who, while recognizing its futility, simply want to do something.

Every day, the staff of the radiation department ex-presses concern for my health. The concern begins when the receptionist asks how I am. Then the nurse who calls my name asks how I am. The radiotherapist who positions me under the table asks how I am and whether I want to see a physician "for any reason." Although Trudie is the technician I see most frequently, often she is busy and another technician helps—turning me on my front, exchanging the set of blocks, asking how I am. Occasionally, I see a doctor in the hallway and he asks how I am. This concern makes me feel creepy. These people want me to be all right so I won't delay the treatment process, holding up their valuable machines and their careful schedules.

My ability to tolerate radiation sickness is not the only uncertainty concerning length of treatment. The physicians have not yet decided whether to radiate my pelvic area—another set of treatments taking an additional six weeks or so. Nor have they decided whether to follow radiation therapy with chemotherapy.

ON MY FIRST THURSDAY, I am weighed, handed a slip, and told to go upstairs. "A lab technician will take your blood." At the same time a woman in her late teens is also sent up for a blood test. Joy introduces herself. She is the first Hodgkin's disease patient I've met. "I guess we're members of the same club," I say.

Joy is a veteran of radiation treatment. She has beautiful long blond hair and she lifts it up to show me her bald spot. "I wept when it began to fall out. I never wept so hard in my life. But it's all right now. It's beginning to grow back."

She tells me that her pelvic area is being irradiated. "Dr. Grey says that I'll probably be sterile. I always wanted to have kids." She tries to say more about her sadness, but can't. She'd cry, but she doesn't have enough energy. I touch her arm. She shudders a little, then pulls herself together. She recommends

a book on Zen. "When I can eat, I'm on a macrobiotic diet."
She wants to give useful advice. "Have you started vomiting yet?" she asks, concerned about me. I haven't. "Oh, you
will, and it'll be awful. I mean, it was awful for me. Once I
started I thought I'd never stop. When you begin vomiting,
remember, relaxation is important. Try to meditate. Try not to
get too upset." She gives me her phone number. "If you freak
out, call me. I'll understand."

For the first time I come into daily contact with cancer
patients, dozens of cancer patients. (The division treats some
five hundred a year.) Together we sit in the basement waiting
room until our names are called. The room is small and narrow. The shape of the walls and the location of the chairs keep
changing due to the constant construction going on, giving the
place the appearance of decay. Frequently, chunks of Sheet-
rock cover the floor and we hear the intermittent sounds of
drills and jackhammers. Torn magazines lie about, full of stale
news and out-of-date fashions, looking as if they have been
read by every other patient in the building before being sent
to the basement.

The room is a jurisdictional no-man's-land. The hospital's
social services department deals with in-patient problems, and
most of us are out-patients. Except for Trudie, the radiation
staff rarely enters the waiting room. Once we cross through
the double doors leading to the machines, we are asked about
our physical health. In the waiting room itself, we patients
rarely talk.

About once a week one of the two linear accelerators
breaks down. Then the waiting room becomes even more
crowded than usual, with not enough chairs for the patients
who have hour-long waits. Breakdowns are routine, because

the high technology equipment is delicate and must meet exacting control standards. The slightest deviation in dosage can be fatal. It is safer and cheaper for us to be treated in the basement, because the machines use millions of volts of direct current.

Every day we look each other over. Everyone has cancer, and every day the radiation makes us sicker. I think of the waiting room as a betting parlor where we wonder, *What are your odds?* Since most of us are out-patients, we have to get dressed to travel to the hospital. Radiation is enervating; few of us give a damn what we look like: we look like hell.

Most women soon stop bothering with makeup or do a sloppy job of it. Skin burn from radiation means that women who usually wear girdles and brassieres stop wearing them. Many women—and some men—have wigs. Some wear them well and will occasionally suggest where to buy them and how to care for them. More often wigs are askew and look grotesque.

The men who initially wore coats and ties to treatment stop doing so. Instead, they wear whatever is convenient—clean or not, pressed or not. Frequently they give up shaving and sprout growths that are not quite beards. Those who still have hair neglect to comb it.

Occasionally a worried parent or friend appears. The outsider stands out, obviously out of place in that room where health and good grooming seem alien.

Usually I stare at my feet, slouched over and waiting for my name to be called. One morning, for some reason, I look up. Standing along the wall is a man in his mid-forties. His hair is combed. His face is shaved. He wears a suit and tie. And his brightly shined wing-tip shoes have laces. Imagine having the energy to tie shoelaces!

I want to look like that. Why can't I wear a freshly pressed shirt and a pinstriped suit? To me he looks like a god.

Then I realize what he is doing here. He is waiting for his wife. She is a fragile, disheveled woman. Her loose-fitting dress is partially unbuttoned revealing telltale purple lines on her skin. I stare again at my shoes.

I have purple lines on my chest and back, which help the technician line up my body under the machine. I am warned to be careful showering. "Don't soap the lines." Even so, about once a week I get fresh lines, because perspiration and bathing fade the dye.

Although Washington's hot, humid weather has already arrived, I am exceedingly modest, never taking off my shirt or even unbuttoning the top buttons when I can avoid it, always sleeping with a top. I hate the purple lines. They stain my sheets and the white silk pajama top from Saks, which Laura bought me while I was in the hospital. The purple lines remind me of the Mark of Cain.

On one of the days when the machine breaks down and we all have to wait for hours, I am sitting on a chair outside my linear accelerator, wearing the ugly green gown. A woman in her early seventies has just changed into her gown and is sitting next to me, waiting for the other, more powerful machine.

A little girl is carried into the room where my linear accelerator is. I know she is a girl because Trudie keeps repeating her name, talking and trying to soothe her. She is maybe three or four years old. Her skin is shriveled up; her brittle twiglike bones jut out. She reminds me of 1960s Biafra posters.

There are purple dye marks on her head and torso. She is crying, trying to pull away from the nurse who is holding and carrying her into the room. I wonder, *If there's a God, how could He allow this to happen?* When the door is locked and the machine begins growling, the woman next to me says, "Why don't they let her die?"

I LATER LEARNED that the little girl had leukemia. Because of the treatment, the chances were good that she would live a long and healthy life. On the other hand, the elderly woman had an advanced case of breast cancer. She was unlikely to survive.

EVERY DAY Charlie, who is about eleven, arrives from Children's Hospital. He wears a football helmet with his name on it. He bends his head down to charge at the patients in the waiting room, using his helmet as a battering ram. The orderly who brings him has a hard time controlling him. "Come on, Charlie. Stop disturbing the nice people. If you're not good, I'll have to tell on you."

Charlie has trouble with his coordination. He can't walk straight and keeps bumping into things. That doesn't stop him from running or, when held, trying to break away. Sometimes Charlie talks to me. Sometimes he rams at my legs while I hold him by the shoulders, laughing. Laughter sounds out of place in that horrible room.

Trudie, who I think is wonderful, compassionate, and surprisingly cheerful, often comes out to get Charlie and carry him into the linear accelerator room. When Charlie sees her, he tries to run away. The orderly then has to catch him, sometimes peeling his arms away from my legs. "Come on, Charlie, you know this isn't going to hurt," the orderly says. "Why don't you let go of the man's leg? You're not acting like a good boy. If you don't behave, you won't get any ice cream this afternoon."

Leaving the building one morning, I meet an ebullient woman in her mid-fifties. We exchange pleasantries until she says, "I have to sit down or I'll collapse." I help her over to a bench. She tells me she is dying. She says that God loves her and she is resigned to dying. "I just want to do it right, that's all. I want to be sure that my children and husband understand. I want them to continue to love God when I die."

Each day becomes more depressing than the last. Because the treatment makes me feel so weak, each day I feel less able to cope with the misery that surrounds me. Sometimes I just sit in the room, staring at my shoes, tears welling up in my eyes, unable to cry. Never before have I experienced so much suffering so consistently. Life might be joy and beauty and happiness for some, but day in and day out I am surrounded by ugliness, sadness, and loss. It doesn't seem fair.

Why do these people have to suffer? Why am I going to live while so many of my fellow patients are going to die? Who makes these terrible decisions? Is it God? Does He know what He is doing? I feel guilty—guilty that I am going to live.

O<small>N THE FIRST DAY</small> of treatment I am exhausted, as if large quantities of blood had been drained out of me. On the second day when Trudie asks how I feel, I say, "Awful. I'm incredibly tired."

She says, "It's unusual for you to feel any side effects this early. Do you want to see a doctor?"

Of course I want to see a doctor. However, I feel that whatever is wrong with me is minor compared to the condition of my fellow patients. Acting out of character I say, "I'll see how I feel tomorrow." I think that doctors have better things to do with their time than take care of my insignificant problem. Perhaps, I think, if I will myself to be strong, I will stop feeling weak.

After treatment the next day, I feel even worse—intensely weak, weepy, tired without any desire for sleep. I ask to see a doctor. Violet leads me past the small closetlike changing room where my clothes are hanging. She says, "Go into the examination room, sit down, and Dr. Diem will be along shortly."

This is the first time I've even heard Dr. Diem's name. Inside the examination room is a pile of Xerox copy lists. At the head of the list it says: "Should you require the attention of one of our physicians at night or on weekends, one of the following doctors will be on call." Although the sheets are clearly intended for patients, I feel furtive as I take one.

Dr. Diem inquires, "What is wrong?"

"I'm exhausted."

"Yes, you might be exhausted. I don't know yet whether the exhaustion is a side effect of the treatment. If you were exhausted a week or two after treatment began, I'd say it was definitely a side effect. But it's a little early for you to be feeling so tired. Do you have trouble swallowing or have a sore throat?"

"No."

Dr. Diem says, "I'm sorry, but there's nothing I can do for you. If you want to see me for any reason, don't hesitate to ask."

The examination is over.

EVERY TIME I entered the division of radiation oncology I felt slightly paranoid. Going back there years after treatment was over—with reporter's notebook in hand—I continued to feel paranoid, even though I knew the machines were turned off for the day and that when tomorrow came I would not be a patient again.

As a patient, my initial polite, diffident behavior—quickly replaced by aggressive, demanding behavior—was phony. Perhaps my behavior was suppressed anger, anger I was afraid to let out for fear of consequences. Perhaps I was transferring my anger onto the division's authority figures, incorrectly assuming that since I was angry at them, they must be angry at me. Or perhaps I felt paranoid because the machines gave me radiation sickness; the bastards really were out to get me.

Patients receiving the same set of treatments I did usually experience, in sequence, sore throat, difficulty swallowing, loss of appetite, malaise, nausea, vomiting, exhaustion, depression, skin burn, and loss of hair. Some do not have all these side effects. I, thank God, didn't vomit. Some have other side effects or experience the usual ones more quickly than expected or more severely. For example, it is relatively uncommon to experience difficulty swallowing after only one or two treatments. In extremely rare cases, however, this side effect can kill the patient.

Radiologists do not know how an individual patient will react to radiation. Some radiologists describe probable side effects to their patients and at what point in treatment to expect them. Others do not want to worry the patients prematurely about what might happen. They are afraid that if a probable side effect is mentioned, then the patient's fear—rather than the radiation itself—might produce the effect psychosomatically.

MY RADIOLOGISTS take the latter approach, which makes me angry. I feel unprepared. I am surrounded by patients experiencing a variety of side effects, which I assume will happen to me. Meanwhile, I am continually asked questions like, "Does your throat hurt?", "Do you feel nauseous?", "Are you vomiting?"

I am angry and frustrated that Dr. Diem is unable to make me feel better. I sit outside Paul's office on Twenty-fourth Street, waiting for morning to turn into afternoon. When group begins I complain about how tired I feel. Then I ask Paul if he can prescribe something that will make me feel better.

"Before I prescribe anything, I want you to talk to your radiologist."

"What could you prescribe?"

"I could give you a prescription for Ritalin, which might make you feel more energetic and lift your spirits. Before I do, I want you to talk to your radiologist to find out whether he thinks it a good idea."

"I've already talked to my radiologist, and he says he doesn't know what's wrong with me."

"Well, I want you to go back to him and tell him that your psychiatrist is willing to prescribe Ritalin for you, but he won't give you a prescription unless he knows whether your exhaustion is a physical reaction or an emotional one. I want to know what causes the side effect before I get involved in treating it."

"Do I have to talk to him again?"

"Yes. Otherwise, I won't give you the prescription."

"But I know what he's going to say. He's going to say that he doesn't know whether I'm crazy or whether it's the fucking machine."

"If you want the prescription," Paul says, "you have to talk to your radiologist first."

That makes me angry, but I swallow my anger and describe a dream I had last night.

I am sitting in a large amphitheater which is either a bullring or a football stadium. Laura and Robert are both there, but they ignore me. I am naked. I try putting on some clothes, which neither belong to me nor fit properly. The clothes are baggy and make me look ridiculous. Also there are several pairs of shoes, waiting to be tried on. The shoes belong to my Italian grandfather, and they are too small. After trying to make them fit, I give up. Meanwhile, Laura and Robert begin leaving the amphitheater. I run after them, calling out their names. They hear me. . . . I awaken just as they turn around.

"What comes to mind," Paul asks, "when you think about your Italian grandfather?"

"I was named after my grandfather. My grandfather is dead. I am supposed to die young, just like my grandfather did."

"Only you're not going to die, are you? You can't fit into his shoes."

I agree that I'm not going to die.

"The dream shows, even before you're willing to admit it consciously, that you no longer feel obliged to relive your grandfather's life. You no longer feel compelled to fit into his shoes or to fit into the whole system that has been making you crazy for all these years. The dream is a recognition that not only are you going to get better physically, but you already are getting better mentally."

He chuckles. "It looks like you're ready to give up being crazy. You're going to have to get used to being emotionally healthy."

I don't like that interpretation at all. Perversely, I don't want anyone, especially my psychiatrist, telling me that I'm not crazy anymore. If he doesn't think I'm crazy, I'll show him!

I should take a cab home. Instead, I decide to suffer.

Paul's office is seven blocks from the subway entrance at Connecticut Avenue. If I were feeling well, I could walk to the subway, take a train, and then transfer to the number 40 bus, which stops in front of my building. Although I'm not feeling well, I do just that—pushing myself too hard.

The short ride from downtown to Union Station is on the first few miles of an ambitious underground mass transportation system still under construction. By the time I arrive at the station, my clothes are drenched in sweat; I am thirsty; I want to climb into bed. I am annoyed that this damn subway has reduced my bus service. A few weeks ago, I could have taken a bus from downtown directly home. The bus no longer goes downtown, and a round trip that used to cost $.80 now costs $1.40.

When I get to the surface, I start looking for the bus stop. I discover that Union Station is in even a worse mess than usual. There's an enormous hole in the middle of the station. After several jurisdictional squabbles among the D.C. city government, the U.S. Department of Interior and the U.S. Department of Transportation, the hole is being converted into a "National Visitors Center" for the Bicentennial. Although there is no way it can be ready in time, Union Station is the site of feverish construction activity on this hot, humid afternoon. Even the circle outside the station is being torn up and repaved. Flagpoles for all fifty states have just been erected, and some flags are flying. No one seems to know the location of the new bus stop, not even the police.

Finally I locate a bus stop, but I'm not sure if it is the right one. A Metro official standing right there doesn't know either. A number 40 bus comes by. The driver stops to let off passengers, but won't let on new ones even though there is room. I become furious, attempting to stand in front of the vehicle so the driver can't get past me. Since he has enough turning room, he swerves around and continues his route. I become absolutely enraged—angrier than I have ever been. I dash across the adjacent park, finding newly discovered strength and energy in my anger.

By foot, the next bus stop—at First and D—is not far. Traffic and a light hold up the driver before he is able to go around the circle and turn right. I reach the stop before the bus. The driver, remembering my previous attempt to stop him, refuses to let me board. Diagonally across the street is a Capitol police station. I again block the bus, but this time the driver cannot get by without running me over.

"Get out of my way."

"Only if you let me on."

"O.K. I'll let you on."

I don't believe him. "Open the door."

Several passengers say, "Come on. Let him in." The door opens.

I attempt to board, but as soon as I get out of his path, the driver again tries to leave without me. Again, I jump out in front of him, and he slams on the brakes.

Several police are going off duty. One calls to me. "What's going on?"

"The driver won't let me on."

The policeman says to the driver, "Let him on."

"O.K. I will," the driver says, and opens the door.

The policeman continues his walk home and does not turn around. As I again attempt to board, the driver guns the accelerator, closing the door and leaving the stop without me.

"You bastard," I yell, pounding at the closing door. The side of my fist hits the top right pane of glass. The rubber mounting, which holds the pane in place, gives way. As the bus moves, the glass falls and shatters. Immediately, the driver stops and puts on the hazard lights.

Another bus comes by. A number 42. It isn't as convenient as a number 40, but it will do. The driver opens to let me on, but I refuse to board and wave him on.

I could cross the street to go into the Monocle Restaurant and order a Coke. But I don't. I am angry. I want to see JUSTICE DONE. I am going to get that son-of-a-bitch bus driver if it is the last thing I do. I stand at the bus stop waiting for the police to get around to arresting me. The cops take their time.

Another off-duty policeman shouts to a colleague in the station, "If they decide to press charges, I'll swear that he broke the window."

The on-duty cop leaves the station and walks over to me. "What's going on?"

"That bastard wouldn't stop for me. Arrest him."

"I didn't see what happened, so I can't arrest him," he says. "Failing to stop for a passenger is not a crime. It's a traffic offense."

"Well, give him a ticket."

"I can't give him a ticket, I didn't see the offense."

Silence. Then he says to me, "Did you break a window in that bus?" The bus is still parked, hazard lights blinking. The door opens.

"No," I say, "I didn't break the bastard's window."

"Wait right here," he says, and walks over to the bus.

He goes inside the bus, talks to the driver, and after a while returns.

"Well," I say belligerently, "are you going to arrest me or not?"

"I don't know yet. I have to find out whether Metro's

going to file a complaint. Why don't you come with me into the station?"

We walk into the station. He suggests that I wait in a small room next to the front desk. I am carrying a birthday present for Laura's son Tim, wrapped in a paper bag. Deciding to make the cops feel really uncomfortable, I take out a pen and start writing everyone's name and badge number on the bag.

Three police forces are involved with my arrest—the Capitol, District of Columbia, and transit police. Physically, I am in the jurisdiction of the Capitol police. They work for Congress, patrolling congressional office buildings and providing police protection for the Capitol and its immediate neighborhood. If they arrest me, I'll be prosecuted by the U.S. Attorney rather than the District government.

However, the Capitol police are not really equipped to keep people in jail. When they arrest someone, they generally use D.C. jails. So, if *they* arrest me, my arresting officer would have to drive me to a District of Columbia police station, which has the facilities for taking my picture, fingerprinting me, and putting me behind bars. The procedure will involve three sets of paper work—the first, charging me with the crime; the second, putting me in the custody of the D.C. police; the third, returning me to the custody of the Capitol police for trial.

Because of the paper work and inconvenience, the Capitol police don't want to arrest me at all. They'd prefer that someone else make the arrest. So they call the transit police. Finally, after twenty minutes, a transit cop and his officer-in-training walk the block and a half from the Union Station subway entrance to the police station. As they look me over, I write down their names. They fiddle with their walkie-talkies, which don't work, then leave the room, looking for a telephone.

The transit police are a force newly created to ensure that D.C. subways and buses do not get the same reputation for crime as New York's. They would like to arrest me. After a telephone call to headquarters, they find out that since I was not inside the bus when I broke the window, I am not within their jurisdiction. However Metro headquarters orders the bus driver, whose fully loaded bus is still across the street, to file a formal complaint against me. I am told that because of a recent wave of vandalism, the bus people are under firm orders to crack down. "I'm sorry," my arresting officer says.

Reluctantly, Officer Calvin Van Hoff reads me my rights. When Officer Bates searches me, I tell him, "Be careful. I just had an operation." He ignores me. When he pats my belly, I howl. I show him my wound and my purple ink marks and ask him to take it easy. He decides that handcuffs are unnecessary.

The charge is Destruction of Private Property. I am charged under the statute, "Destroying or defacing buildings, statues, monuments, offices, dwellings, and structures." Maximum penalty is six months in jail and one hundred dollars fine.

I ask whether I can call my lawyer. I can and do. Ernest Lockwood, who does legal work for Washington Independent Writers, tells me not to worry. "You'll be out on bail shortly. Call me if you have any problems. Say nothing about your case."

It is 3:30. I ask Van Hoff, "Will I be out in time to take my lady friend and her son out for dinner?" Van Hoff says yes and lets me use the phone again. I call Laura, telling her that I am in jail.

She is angry. "What have you done this time?"

171

"I'm talking over a police telephone and I haven't done anything, not this time nor at any time. I'm calling to let you know that I may be delayed, but that Officer Van Hoff assures me I'll be out in time to take you and Tim to dinner." I am angry at her, which causes me to express myself in a formal, stilted manner. I'm angry that she even thinks I've done something wrong, and I'm angry that she's not being more supportive.

Two hours after breaking the window, I am wiping the fingerprint ink off my fingers. I am asked about permanent scars. I show the officer Dr. Simpson's handiwork. I am asked about on-going medical treatment. If I am unable to make bail, then—according to procedure—a police doctor has to be informed of my radiation treatment; he, then, has to decide whether my medical treatment should be continued. I have images of being transported to G.W. Hospital in a paddy wagon, sitting in the division of radiation oncology waiting room handcuffed to a policeman!

As I wait in the holding cell, several policemen come over, asking about my cancer. They try to reassure me. One says, "This is a chickenshit charge. Don't worry about it." I pay no attention to the reassurances and worry a lot.

The computerized FBI check comes up negative. The desk officer at Fifth and E, S.E. calls Robert, whom I've listed as my character reference. He talks to Robert at work—the men's furnishings department of the Georgetown University Shop. "This is Patrolman Ramsay, at the District of Columbia Police Department, First Substation. One Joel Ezra Solkoff is under arrest and he gave your name as a reference. Do you know Mr. Solkoff? Does he reside at _____ ? How long has he lived at that address? What is his present occupation?

Do you know of any reason why his release might be a danger to the health and safety of the District of Columbia? Thank you for your help."

The procedure for bail is simple. Since I am not on the wanted lists of the D.C. police or the FBI and my crime is sufficiently petty, I can be released on my own recognizance. That means no bail costs, with my own "good name" as guarantee.

I am out in plenty of time for dinner. Carrying a Citation to Appear at the Criminal Division of the District of Columbia Superior Court (U.S. attorney cases) on July 2, 1976, I hail a cab right outside the police station. Home is a few blocks away, but I am too exhausted to walk. I have been one *CLASS A IDIOT*, and knowing that is no comfort.

THE DAY is not over yet. Of course I'm tired and want to cancel dinner with Laura and Tim. But canceling is more complicated than going through with it. The children are now living for the summer at their father's house in Maryland. Laura has already arranged to pick up Tim and arrangements between Laura and her former husband are stressful. My canceling and rescheduling will raise the general anxiety level and consequently the anxiety level between Laura and me. I am too tired to even consider doing that. I figure that nothing can make this horrible day worse.

I call Laura and tell her I am out of jail. She says, "Tim wants to eat at Blackie's."

"That's fine with me. Tim should decide where he wants to go for his birthday dinner."

Blackie's House of Beef has showcases of guns, Wild West souvenirs, and political bric-a-brac. Near the bar is a machine typing out the latest news from one of the wire services. When we enter, Hubert Humphrey is standing next to the register talking on the cashier's telephone and simultaneously shaking hands. Humphrey, there for dinner, is enjoying a burst of public affection. His return to popularity is largely a reaction to Jimmy Carter, whose nomination is virtually assured. The press is printing scenarios of the Democratic convention turning to its "elder statesman." The scenarios are absurd because of the delegate count, but the feeling of nostalgia and affection for Humphrey is widespread, and Blackie's customers are delighted to see him.

I have interviewed Humphrey, who is a member of the Senate Agriculture Committee, and I've covered his confrontations with Earl Butz. I introduce Laura and Tim to the senator. Laura, torn between a hatred for politicians and a schoolgirl love for celebrities, is impressed. Tim is excited because he's seen Humphrey on television. During dinner, Tim keeps asking the name of "that famous man" so he can tell his brother and sister.

About ten minutes after we order, the conversation becomes quiet. Laura is angry at me. Among other things she is angry that I was arrested. Neither of us wants to talk about that in front of Tim. What would Jim say? So our communication is strained. Meanwhile Tim is suspicious of my motives.

Dinner represents my first attempt to restore contact with the children. It was planned immediately after my release from the hospital, when I was still full of frenetic energy. I thought that doing something for the children would be a good way of making Laura happy, of paying her back for all the things she did for me. I thought that Tim's birthday would be a handy excuse to begin a round of events with the children designed to deal with their fears of my sickness and to let them know I still cared about them. Tonight, however, I feel too tired, depressed, and full of self-pity to deal with the present, let alone think of the future. All I want is for Laura to hold me—although her disapproval is so strong that I'll settle for sulking alone in my apartment.

Previously Tim and I had gone out together alone. This time he wants his mother with him, and that angers me. How am I going to reach Tim if he uses Laura as a barrier between us? Of course Tim is afraid of my cancer and of relating to me, and I, too, am full of my own fears. I am not up to dealing with a hostile nine-year-old who is afraid of me.

I make perfunctory efforts to talk to Tim, but he is not interested. When I say good-night, mumbling, "We're going to have to get together soon," I am all too aware that dinner was a failure.

Before driving Tim to Maryland Laura drops me off at her house, which is on the way. She doesn't want Jim to see me. As I get out, Tim turns to his mother, "Does *he* have a key?"

"No, he doesn't have a key."

As I am waiting outside the door for Laura to return, I feel like one of her children and realize how detrimental this is to any relationship, especially ours. I resent her children and feel humiliated by my resentment.

Later, lying with Laura in the king-size bed Jim bought, I feel angry and depressed that I am not strong enough to be the man she wants and needs.

17

SOMETIMES I FELT that the world did not exist outside of me, my health, my doctors, my trips to the radiation room, and my relationships. Unless I stayed alive, the world could not continue. The world owed me. When I felt miserable, I had the right to impose my feelings on others.

My rage, my breaking the window and getting caught, made me see that an outside reality existed. No matter how much I wanted it to, having cancer didn't exempt me from the same rules required of healthy people. It didn't give me license to break bus windows or the law. Getting arrested taught me that there were clear limits to my conduct. Unfortunately, it took me a while to learn that lesson.

THE NEXT DAY, Friday, June 25, after radiation for that day and the week is over, Violet tries to discourage me from bothering the doctor again. "Of course, if there's something else wrong . . ." When Dr. Diem sees me for the second day in a row for the same complaint, he is polite, but his tone implies that I am a pest.

I anticipate what he is going to say, and Paul's requirement that I hear him out irritates me. Dr. Diem says, "As I told you yesterday, there's nothing I can do for your symptoms of exhaustion."

"My psychiatrist is willing to give me Ritalin."

"I didn't know you were seeing a psychiatrist." He makes it sound like an accusation.

"My psychiatrist won't give me Ritalin unless you agree that it's all right for me to have it. He wants to know whether my exhaustion is biological or psychological."

Dr. Diem tells me again that he doesn't know what causes my exhaustion. Exhaustion is a biological side effect of treatment; it is early for me to be experiencing exhaustion as a side effect; some patients experience side effects earlier than others.

"So, it's all right with you if Dr. Weisberg gives me Ritalin?"

"Yes, I have no objection. However, it might be a good idea for you to wait a while and see what happens. If you continue to feel tired, then you can start taking the drug."

"I don't want to wait. Do you have any objection if my psychiatrist gives me the stuff right now?"

He doesn't, but it takes him a while to say so.

I go directly to Paul's office, waiting for a break between appointments so he can write out a prescription. I am too short-tempered to say thank you.

I am annoyed because I want energy. I want it instantly, and I am willing to try anything to make me feel better. I am angry at Dr. Diem and at Paul for making me go through this medical rigmarole. If some fucking prescription has some chance of making me feel better, then why don't they just give it to me without all this bullshit?

At first, the Ritalin makes me feel a little peppier. But as the weeks of radiation treatment continue, nothing affects the overwhelming sense that all energy has left my body.

I am taking twenty mg of Ritalin a day. I want more. At one group session, I add to my list of complaints the fact that Paul's fucking Ritalin isn't doing me any good. "What happens if I increase the dosage?"

Paul says, "I'd advise against it. What you're taking now is fine. Substantial increases in dosage can cut off oxidation to the brain, presenting the risk of brain damage."

I heed Paul's advice.

ON SATURDAY, I go to my lawyer's office in a seedy building at Fourteenth and G. The only working elevator wheezes as it slowly ascends. In the waiting room, I hear through the thin glass partition Lockwood talking in a tone intended to calm and reassure. I hope his voice will have the same tone with me.

Lockwood apologizes for keeping me waiting.

I explain, "If that son-of-a-bitch bus driver had picked me up, this whole thing never would have happened. He's the one who should have been arrested, not me."

He points out that the driver did not commit a misdemeanor. "However, if it comes to trial, the jury might be sympathetic."

"Anyway," I say, "it's not my fault the window broke. I didn't hit it hard enough to break it. The fault was Metro's. If they had mounted the window more securely, it never would have fallen out and broken. Why should I be responsible because the bus company doesn't install its windows properly?"

"You set in motion the chain of events that led to the breaking of the window. Therefore, you are responsible for breaking the window, whether you did so directly or indirectly."

"It's not fair," I grumble. I'm combative because that's one way—certainly not an attractive way—I deal with fear. I'm afraid of lawyers' fees, court appearances, fines, jail, and the embarrassment of being publicly exposed as an asshole.

He says, "I don't think it will go to the trial stage. Metro will probably drop the complaint or fail to appear. If they fail to appear enough times, I can make a motion to drop the case. That can take several months. If it does go to trial, the jury is likely to let you off. For this kind of offense, D.C. juries are generally lenient, but I wouldn't count on that if I were you. Since you don't have a record, you almost certainly will not go to jail. The worst you can expect is a fine and a suspended sentence."

Lockwood recommends that I go to the first court appearance without him. "It will be a waste of your money and my time for me to go. If Metro does pursue the complaint, and if the U.S. attorney does decide to prosecute, then we can decide what to do next."

I don't like that.

"I'll go," he agrees, "but you'll have to pay me for my time."

I give him a check for fifty dollars, thinking it unfair that this whole mess should actually be costing me money.

He says, "I'll call your arresting officer. Since he didn't actually see the offense, maybe he'll think that it's not worth his time to keep coming back to court." We talk about my cancer. He says, "Maybe, the officer will be sympathetic about your disease."

I say, "I don't want to use my disease to get out of this."

Neither of us believes me.

ALL WEEK LONG I have a series of short unpleasant dreams about jail and closed rooms, but yesterday when Robert asked about the court appearance, I joked about it. Last night, even though the air conditioner made the apartment frigid, I awoke in the middle of the night sweating. I kicked off the covers, trying to forget the image of me at age two and a half. In the dream, I am in the lower sleeping compartment of a train. The curtain is drawn, and I am naked and sweating, being taken away from home. The train's movement sounds like the jangling of a jailer's keys.

On Friday morning, July 2, I am at courtroom A-317, building A, Criminal Division, Superior Court, Fifth and E streets, N.W.—just as it says on my Citation to Appear. I am here exactly at 9:00, ignoring Lockwood's advice. He told me, "It isn't necessary to be there at nine because the judge doesn't leave chambers until nine-thirty or ten."

I am wearing a suit. The bailiff tries to seat me with the lawyers. Forty-five minutes later Lockwood peers at me in the courtroom, motioning for me to join him outside, saying, "Look, I talked to the arresting officer and to the U.S. attorney. They're going to drop the charges. The whole thing is over." He smiles. "You can relax now. Congratulations. However, you can't leave right now, otherwise you'll forfeit bail. You've got to stay until your name is called. When it's called, the judge will tell you that you can go. You don't need me for this. Is it all right with you if I leave now?"

It isn't all right with me, but I don't say so. His office

might be shabby, but Lockwood clearly knows what he's doing. True, I want someone to hold my hand (so to speak). But I know that isn't necessary. So I wait alone, listening to the dismal roll call. One man is arraigned for stealing a pair of shoes. At the bench in front of me, two lawyers are discussing how much to charge for a first-degree murder case.

Finally, my name is one of twenty called for "failure to prosecute." The bailiff lines us all up in front of the judge, making sure our names match his list. My mates are all black. I am the only defendant the judge calls Mister when he tells us we are free to go.

I don't feel grateful for being let off. Instead, I luxuriate in anger at the criminal justice system and at my conviction that fellow victims of the system who are poor and black aren't released as easily as I. I feel guilty for being free. I interrupt these thoughts to remind myself—self-pityingly—that I am now free to go to radiation. Leaving the courtroom, I feel as if the incident never happened, that it was a bad dream best forgotten.

Several weeks later, Aaron mentions that my arresting officer called him. Aaron is amused, calling me "jailbird." "Shut up," I tell him, annoyed and surprised, as if the event took place years ago, and how could he be so rude as to remind me of it? I don't feel grateful to Aaron, to the policeman who went out of his way for me, or to Lockwood who simplified the whole mess. I feel put upon by the notion that I ought to be held accountable for my actions. *Fuck everybody. I have cancer.*

MEANWHILE, on Tuesday, June 29, before the scheduled court appearance, I tell group about the arrest. I describe it in the bland matter-of-fact tone of one recalling last week's not very interesting picnic. The telling takes at least twice as long as necessary, as I detail the police jurisdictional problems and describe the stations in which I was held. The group is again shocked into unaccustomed silence.

Then Paul says, "It's a classic example of negative reaction to a positive dream interpretation. Last week I tell you that you are getting better. On the same day, you go out and do something stupid just to show me how crazy you are. I ought to write it up and send it to a journal."

Changing his mood, Paul laughingly asks, "What do you think of when you think of a bus?"

I say, "Buses are large, necessary, unreliable, secure . . . A few years ago I wasn't paying attention and crashed my bicycle into a bus that stopped suddenly . . . When I lived in California, I had an affair with a woman who lived in a school bus. She was artistic. Later I found out she was slightly crazy . . ."

"Who in your life does a bus remind you of?"

"My mother." I sneer contemptuously. "I knew you were leading to that."

Jack comments on the humdrum way I described the incident. "It's as if, even now, you're afraid to express your rage. When you were a child and you expressed anger at your mother, is that how you felt? Were you afraid of your own anger, trying to dry out your rage by pretending it didn't exist? Your detailed description of that first room, where you waited for the police to formally charge you—you make it sound almost as if you were glad you were there. Being arrested has all the attractions of being with mother. It is womblike, all-encompassing; everything is taken care of for you."

Paul says angrily, "You wanted to be arrested. Why the hell didn't you get out of there after you broke the window?

You could have taken another bus. You could have walked across the street. Instead, you just stood there waiting to be arrested. Why are you so self-destructive and crazy that you go out of your way to be arrested?"

I become indignant. I complain that it was the bus driver's fault, not mine, and I wanted to have the police arrest *him*—to see justice done. I complain that the group doesn't care about me, that shrinks see Mother in everything, that I don't feel well . . .

After a while, I get tired of listening to myself speak, but I'm angry, especially at Paul.

Paul says, "Are you done?"

I snarl, "Yes, I'm done."

"I want the group to tell you what they think. Doris?"

Doris turns to me, "I don't know what to say. It makes me really sad. I pity you that you feel so bad the only way you can express it is by breaking a window and getting arrested."

Sally says, "It frightens me. I didn't realize you have all that rage inside you."

Lois says, "You just want some attention. I'm annoyed that you don't ask for it directly."

PAUL LATER SAID, "When you were crazy and pounding on the bus and demanding to make your presence known, that came directly out of a fear of dissolution, a fear that your being would be unacknowledged and through being unacknowledged would be unreal."

In other words, I still had not come to terms with my fear of death. Even though I knew rationally that I was not going to die, emotionally I was still afraid. Breaking the bus window was a way of acting out my fear of death.

Paul defined death as ceasing to be, dissolution, saying,

"The last time that ceasing to be is a great threat is in early childhood." The issue of "ceasing to be" is only recently understood. Within the past few decades psychiatric researchers—working in an area neglected by Freud—have demonstrated the importance of early childhood on personality development, when some infants turn to the wall and die. This phenomenon, called "failure to thrive," occurs even though the infants are physically healthy and adequately nourished. They die, researchers found, because they are neglected emotionally—are not loved.

According to Paul, my breaking the bus window and the fear of death that it demonstrated related directly back to personality development in infancy. An infant who turns to the wall and dies does so because he does not feel connected, does not feel whole. As a young man in my twenties, the last time I had experienced the fear of death in any meaningful way was in early infancy, when I feared that I would not get enough love and would just dissolve, cease to be.

The popular notion that disease victims do better if they want to live relates to this fear of dissolution. Something about the disease process and the frightening, exhausting treatments for cancer often cause patients to act like children. Childlike behavior is a return to simpler, basic feelings toward major emotional issues, a process psychiatrists call "regression." Regression, while it may not be attractive, is certainly understandable. If the patient's basic feelings about himself and the world—formulated during early childhood—are fundamentally sound, then there is no cause for alarm.

My feelings about myself and the world—formulated during early childhood—were not basically sound. During my infancy, Mother went through a series of emotional crises.

Although I was not a failure-to-thrive infant, Paul explained, "During the first three years of your life your mother was often unavailable to you, and when she was available her love was inconsistent. Those are the years when the primary bond between mother and child is broken and an autonomy occurs in the healthy person. That autonomy did not happen with you, and you maintained a yearning for the kind of closeness that had not occurred when it should have occurred." Therefore, I remained vulnerable to feelings of abandonment and dissolution.

Ideally, mothers who are secure with themselves reward their children for autonomous behavior, letting the child know that he is loved when he leaves mother to walk, play, and explore his surroundings. Some mothers find this period of separation especially difficult, being afraid to let go of a bond that keeps mother and child as one. The mother reacts by rewarding the child for dependent behavior and punishing for independent behavior. Fathers of these children worsen the problem by being passive and encouraging dependency. The result is a child who is not secure within himself, who grows older finding within himself the natural desire to be independent, but feeling anxious and frighteningly incomplete when he tries to lead his own life. His behavior may be overtly dependent or combatively independent (apparently rejecting the tie that binds). Either way, he has difficulty dealing with work, love, friendship.

Paul explained, "In your late twenties, without ever considering this as an issue (because people don't know what's bothering them) you got yourself into psychotherapy with a doctor who recognized the problem."

Before the cancer, I was making considerable progress in

therapy identifying and dealing with my problem. Paul feared that I would allow my disease to undo that progress and return me to a state of emotional dependency.

Paul later said that his initial reaction to my cancer diagnosis was, "Oh, shit. I was afraid of regression more than death. I mean I knew that you might die. But I knew that with modern methods you were not likely to die this year. So, the prime issue causing my 'Oh, shit' reaction was the effect the cancer could have on any tendency to regress back to your mother's arms."

I suspect that one reason Paul wanted me to tell Mother about the cancer was to forestall my feelings of dependency. By dealing with her while I was still feeling relatively well, I would find it more difficult to lean on her during the expected radiation-caused depression. Much of my psychological difficulty was caused, after all, by my still dealing with my mother as a symbol. I was not treating her as a twenty-eight-year-old man treats a fifty-one-year-old woman who happens to be his mother. Instead, I was relating to her as MOTHER, with the symbolism and emotional charge that had been applicable and useful when I was an infant. Fighting with Mother in the hospital, refusing to give in to her wishes to care for me even though I yearned to be cared for had managed—however unpleasantly—to check a serious threat to my emotional independence. However that threat was not necessarily over. Among other things, refusal to give in to my actual mother didn't prevent me from creating a series of symbolic mothers—buses, police departments, psychiatrists, or Laura.

The combination of my operation, wound infection, radiation, and fear of additional cancer treatment made me feel like one of the walking dead. The rage at the bus *(Goddamn you, bus, you're going to stop or else)* was a way of proving to myself that I was alive, that I was a member of the angry, dissatisfied, pissed-off living rather than the complaisant, passive, well-behaved dying. But behaving destructively—primarily self-destructively—was not a good sign. I still had rotting, unexpressed feelings waiting to bubble to the surface surrounded by infection and pus, like one of those sutures Simpson left in my gut.

18

THE MOST SURPRISING side effect of radiation therapy is that I really have no appetite. I don't want food. The smell makes me nauseous. I am never hungry. The thought of eating makes me queasy.

I've always been a compulsive eater, eating whether hungry or not—just for the sake of eating. Suddenly food is totally repulsive. At first, lack of appetite seems a bonus. I lose the ten pounds that, off and on since college, I needed to lose.

Every day I have to make a conscious effort to eat. If I don't eat, the radiation will make me even weaker. Then they'll have to stop the radiation, wait for me to get stronger, and start again, lengthening the treatment process.

I soon abandon any attempt to concern myself with nutrition—not that my physicians ever mention the subject. My primary objective is to force as many calories inside as possible in the least repulsive manner. Frequently, on trips back from downtown or when friends bring over food, I get a Sara Lee pound cake. If I am patient and force myself, I can eat an entire cake at one sitting. The odor is not offensive and the taste is all right. I also can drink Cokes. At 120 calories a glass, they help fatten me up.

The less time I spend with food, the easier it is to eat. I am acutely sensitive to odor. I avoid anything that smells like food. I am finicky. Food has to be bland. I often examine it like a two-year-old unwilling to eat anything new or unpleasant looking. By working hard enough at it, I am able to eat the equivalent of two meals a day.

At first I try to get downtown early to eat before the radiation makes me sicker and more nauseous. But the odor in the hospital corridor is so overpowering that I soon have to give up on breakfast.

Lunch frequently involves sitting at a bar nursing a Coke. Although I am unable to tolerate liquor, I sit at the bar because bars are usually located away from the kitchen. If the Coke goes down without much difficulty I order soup, and then if I still don't feel too queasy, a sandwich.

For dinner I frequently force myself to walk four blocks to Duddington's, which has an inexpensive steak-and-salad menu. I go early when the place is still empty and I can choose a seat close to the exit. I order London broil (without sauce) and pay my check before the food comes. Then, after going to the salad bar, I race to put enough food inside before being overcome with nausea.

Late one afternoon Congressman Peter Rodino sits next to me. I want to ask him how it feels to impeach a president. Instead prudence requires that I make a quick getaway.

Soon radiation therapy becomes my entire life. Every day it becomes harder to get up, get dressed, and go downtown for more. Since my energy is severely limited, I need to make sure that I have enough of it to get to G.W. and back. Some days I have to start earlier so I don't exhaust myself in rushing. Some days I have to take a cab home because I just can't make it otherwise.

"TODAY IS a good day for me," I write my friend David. "It's a late Sunday afternoon, and I feel alive. My mind is not in a spacy radiation fog, and for the first time since I was hospitalized it seems I'm likely to finish something—this letter to you. A month of half-starts has been a bummer."

Each week, as I get closer to 3,963 rads—the level required to complete the first round—the radiation sickness gets worse. At first I can look forward to the weekends. Even though each weekday is harder than the last, during the weekend pause in treatment I feel a temporary return of energy. But after several weeks the pause no longer provides relief.

"Friday was the day my hair started to fall out in huge clumps," I write to David. "Each clump could easily fill up a flat-bottomed champagne glass. Last week the clumps only had about 15 hairs and could be contained in a small locket. Friday I also got cream for my radiation burn; like sunburn, it gives me that healthy glow. Fuck. Also, Thursday I began feeling nauseated and squeamish about eating. I started to have that horrid feeling that each meal I eat I will not hold. Plus it hurts to swallow."

LAURA REMEMBERED the day my hair fell out: "We were at Dan and Nora's house in Kensington. Your friend Arthur was there. We had just come from seeing *The Big Bus*, which was a silly movie. Arthur was being his pain-in-the-ass self, as he usually is, whining about his wife and about life in general. You were just sitting there. You were quiet, too quiet, and you

190

were real thin. You put your hand to the back of your head, taking out huge tufts of hair and showing them to me. I said to myself, *I'm not going out with a bald man. I hate bald men.* I felt sorry for you because," she said with a laugh, "your hair is your crowning glory. I mean you have such nice hair. You like your hair, and I thought it was awful that it was falling out. It was scary. It was just another thing that was going to be difficult."

Laura's son Luke remembered: "When you got radiation you didn't look very good. All you did was sit around. When you came over we didn't do anything. You just came over.

"You were cranky a lot. A couple of times you'd get mad over little things like the cats running around the house. My mother wanted to put them in the basement. I remember once you jumped on the cat. You dived down on it. We were really mad that you did that.

"I guess it's real mean, but when your hair fell out I thought it looked real funny. I noticed that you were bald up to the back of your head. You couldn't see it all that well, unless you turned a certain way. I think I asked my mother, 'Is Joel's hair always going to be like that? Is he going to be bald?' I guess I was worried you'd be bald like that for the rest of your life. You weren't bald the way most people get bald, because no one gets bald there. Whenever I saw it it made me feel sad about the disease and everything."

BICENTENNIAL DAY is a big deal. The town has been preparing for over a year. Even the agriculture department has put out a special red-white-and-blue bicentennial yearbook. Vice President Nelson Rockefeller is going to lead a parade downtown. Special fireworks are promised.

It is one of those rare Washington July days when the

weather is not unbearably muggy. Past my apartment, hundreds of people are streaming down the sidewalk toward the Capitol. The Capitol has a good view of the parade route and a great view of the mall, where the fireworks will be shot off. All day long, excited clusters of happy people, waving flags and carrying picnic baskets and coolers, are sauntering down East Capitol Street.

The obvious happiness of others makes me angry and despondent. How dare they have a good time when I'm sick? Inside, I close the drapes and turn on the television. Walter Cronkite is euphoric about the Tall Ships entering New York harbor. I switch to an independent station and watch reruns of bad movies. I do not want to be involved in this event.

Laura is scheduled to pick me up for dinner. She's made a reservation at a Marriott motel in Virginia so we can see the fireworks from the rooftop restaurant. The parade causes a traffic jam, and she is two hours late.

I call the Marriott. The maitre d' has given our reservations to someone else. I ask whether his restaurant has a view of the fireworks. "No, you are thinking of _____" Laura made reservations at the wrong Marriott.

She suggests going to the right one. It is late. It will take forever to get across town. The place will certainly be crowded. Tired and pissed off, I tell Laura, "I'm not hungry anyway. I don't want to see the fireworks. I'm going to bed."

LAURA LATER SAID, "God, that was a terrible night. I was all worn out trying to please you. It must have been indicative of my emotional condition that so many things went wrong. I felt like an ass."

I GET A LOT from Laura. I get her love and companionship. On the nights she comes over, I await her arrival, feeling secure that soon she will be with me. I want her to tell me about her day—about her office, children, relatives, and cats. I find that touching her is wonderful. Because of radiation burn—sensitive red patches on my chest, shoulders, and back— even brushing up against someone on the bus is painful and repulsive. However, touching Laura makes me feel whole.

Despite Aaron's prediction that I would be impotent, I'm not. Sex is now my only pleasure. I don't know where I find the energy, but unlike everything else in life which is distasteful or drab, sex is the only thing that makes me feel good. It gives me hope that life's other pleasures will return. It also helps give me a sense of dignity, because I can satisfy her.

BEFORE THE CANCER, I often marveled at Laura's ability to maintain her hectic pace. I told her frequently how much I admired that ability, but after a while I took it for granted. That was how she lived. It never occurred to me that my illness and its demands might be beyond Laura's capacity. I assumed she would manage to juggle me into her busy schedule and do so admirably.

We never seriously talked about the practical difficulties of my care. The only planning I did took place before the operation, when I was capable of caring for myself. At the time, I assumed that the hospital would take care of my postoperative care. I figured that when I was released, I might need a few days rest, but that would be all. Concerning treatment, when I thought of it at all, I assumed that I'd be one of those strong-willed men—like Hubert Humphrey or the examples the doctors told me about—who refused to let radiation or chemotherapy interfere with their daily routine.

Laura was also unprepared. The cancer was not simply an additional difficulty in our relationship, it changed the dynamics between us. My mother's visit, for example, made it obvious that my family was no longer a factor in my relationship with Laura.

On one level, the cancer made us closer. It made me realize that Laura was the most important person in my life. Confronted with the value of life itself, I felt that Laura made it worth living.

That might have overcome all difficulties, but it didn't. My operation and the radiation treatments made me physically and emotionally weak. I felt rotten and dependent upon Laura. As I continued to feel worse, I needed her more. *Her* needs, however, I ignored. I did not raise her spirits and give her the support that made being together worth her while. Frequently she wondered how much longer she was going to do all the giving.

It was clearly necessary for us to talk about ourselves and our future together. But we didn't. I didn't talk because I was too absorbed in myself to realize that talking was necessary. "I didn't talk to you about how I felt," she later told me, "because I was so physically and emotionally exhausted. I was angry at you and I was afraid of expressing my anger. I was angry, among other things, because you were constantly complaining and because you failed to appreciate how much effort I put into caring for you in the hospital. Also, I guess, there was another reason why I was angry. This doesn't sound very nice, but I was angry that you were going to die, and I didn't want you to leave me."

ON WEDNESDAY, July 14, returning from radiation therapy, I can barely make it upstairs. I lie in bed staring at the clumps of my hair that litter the bedroom floor. There is enough hair to fill half a pillow, but I don't have the energy to sweep it up.

I know I should eat, but I don't have the energy to go out. There is a phone on the night table. After leafing through the Yellow Pages I make several calls, but can't find a grocery store or restaurant that will deliver.

I call Robert at the University Shop. Someone there says he is busy. When Robert calls back, I tell him I am hungry. "Will you get me a sandwich?"

"Look, I'm on the other side of town and can't leave work right now. Is it an emergency?"

"No," I say, "it isn't an emergency." I am angry that Robert doesn't drop everything and come over.

Then I call Laura. "I'll come by at the end of the day and bring you a sandwich. Why? Do you need it right away?"

"No, that's all right," I say, feeling abandoned.

I reach for the book at the night table—*Blood Sport* by Dick Francis. I've already read it. "I awoke with foreboding . . ." the book begins. "Slowly relaxing, I turned half over and squinted at the room. A quiet, empty, ugly room. One third of what for want of a less cozy word I called home." Three more times I read about a detective who is nearly suicidal because he was forced to retire as a jockey. I am too tired to get out of bed and get another book. My eyes keep tearing and I feel miserably alone and sad.

Laura arrives at 5:45. "I'm between errands. The kids are waiting for me and I'm late. Matthew asked Olin to get you a sandwich and something to drink." She hands me a paper bag.

I unwrap a tunafish sandwich. The white bread is coated with mayonnaise. The drink is a thick chocolate shake. It's warm and the thick corn-syrup sweetness makes me gag. I throw the food across the room. "This stuff is shit! I can't eat this!"

LATER, LAURA SAID, "When you threw the sandwich across the room, I knew that part of it was that you didn't think you were getting enough attention. Maybe you weren't, but I just couldn't do everything you wanted."

Throwing the food was another example of my fight with reality. By not having asked for help earlier, by not using the little energy I did have to make sure that I ate, I had so increased my dependency that it became unendurable. I had moved beyond exhaustion and beyond the need for food into a state of pure rage. Laura did not love me enough, otherwise why would she bring me such unappetizing food and bring it so late. My friends didn't love me enough, otherwise why were they neglecting me and my needs. My behavior was literally infantile. I was angry. I was needy. I felt self-pity. I threw a temper tantrum like a six-month-old baby whose bottle was late.

ON THURSDAY, I complain to group about the shitty tunafish sandwich.

Paul gets angry. "Listen, if you need help, all you have to do is ask for it. Yesterday, all you really had to do was call my office. Martie [his secretary] would be glad to get you a sandwich and bring it over by cab. You could have called anyone in this group. Anyone here would be delighted to come over and bring you food." One by one he polls each of the group members. Each agrees. He says, "We'd much rather help you than listen to you complain all the time."

Twice a week, Tuesdays and Thursdays, I have to go to group. The distance between group and radiation is close enough that I can combine trips. Group helps me put the cancer experience into perspective. It gives me a place where I can be myself without being pampered—a place where I can realize that other people have problems too.

DORIS REMEMBERED: "You looked awful. I couldn't understand how you got the energy to come to group and why you even bothered. You were thin and you looked like you were going to die. I felt really worried for you. When you came, all you did was complain."

Jack said, "That was a grim period."

Lois told me, "I remember you were complaining all the time. You talked about your apartment being dirty and how all those newspapers were there and how you didn't have the energy to wash the dishes or do any work. I said that if I heard about how dirty your apartment was one more time I'd scream."

LAURA TOLD ME AFTERWARD, "I do remember being angry at you, not being able to express it, but being angry. You were an extremely difficult person to be around, but I persevered just the same. I had the feeling that it wasn't worth it after a while. Sometimes it seemed like nothing I could do could please you. If I did something it would only take care of one thing and you'd have another complaint. I really do think that you had determined that I was the person who was supposed to take care of you, and that meant that I was just supposed to do everything you wanted and do it right and make you feel better. I resented that. I felt trapped."

IT IS JULY 1981. Yesterday, my fiancée Diana and I rented a truck, cornered some friends into helping us, and moved in together. We are sitting at the butcher-block table at our new apartment, staring at a view of 1890s rooftops.

Diana wants me to stop thinking about my five-year-old cancer experience and a love that did not succeed. "Concentrate on me and our wedding plans," she says. "You asked too much of Laura," she says, dismissing the subject.

IT HAD NOT OCCURRED TO ME that I asked more of Laura than she was willing or able to give. For a long time I was perplexed over what went wrong. I assumed that it was my fault—that somehow during the cancer experience I had failed her. But, it was no one's fault.

That summer Laura was unwilling to move in with me, even though the children were with their father. She had reasons, but it took me years to realize that her reasons were a way of avoiding action. Laura wouldn't share her life with me, or couldn't. More precisely, Laura didn't want to share in my life. She thought that I was dying and felt sorry for me. She cared for me as best she could and resented me for it. Laura was trapped because she loved me.

That summer of 1976, money is even scarcer than before, and I am getting desperate. The lawyer in New York wisely decides to settle and the consulting job disappears. My health insurance is all screwed up. I keep getting dunning letters from the hospital and my doctors. Somehow I manage to deal with the paperwork and the bureaucrats at Blue Cross and get the whole mess straightened out. But it is demoralizing. I borrow money from everyone in sight and it still isn't enough.

The article on the USDA for *The Washingtonian* magazine is already several months late. I sit at the typewriter, too weak to lift my fingers to strike the keys. After considerable uncoordinated effort—having to unstick the keys and force my fingers to move to the right places—I am unable to complete a thought. Why do I want this sentence here? What am I trying to say? How long will the article be? How should the paragraphs be arranged? Do I have enough information? Trying to confront the task one step at a time, I return to the sentence I am trying to type. I give up, frustrated, pounding the typewriter with my fist. I am overwhelmed.

The fact that I have something I need to do (write an article) gives me something to aspire to. However, on many days I can only work for ten minutes before my ability to concentrate completely disappears. Then I watch reruns of "Star Trek" on Channel 20, or reread the Horatio Hornblower books and countless murder mysteries. I am too weak to do anything else, but not tired enough to sleep all day as well as all night. I need to have something to keep my mind occupied without challenging it.

I find I can't read a book I haven't read before. I have to be familiar with the characters, style, and plot or else the book is meaningless. Similarly, I find it difficult to watch television programs that aren't reruns.

Finally, by some miracle, the article is done. "To be fair," it says, "the Department of Agriculture was a boring and useless place even before John Ehrlichman hired Earl Butz. President Nixon made it possible for Butz to turn it into the most scandal-ridden department in USDA's history." The article is cranky and crochety, in keeping with the magazine's reputation and my mood. It is full of offbeat details. However, it doesn't have any structure. What I hand in is a working draft, badly in need of a rewrite.

When I go to see Jack Limpert, the editor, he says, "Your main point seems to be that you don't like the Department of Agriculture." I ask Limpert for advice on how to change it. He gives me a lecture on professionalism.

I leave his office feeling like weeping, which is no way for a free-lance writer to feel. Diatribes from angry editors are an occupational hazard even when they're not deserved. I react as if Limpert has criticized my very existence. So I send him a letter. "I am undergoing radiation treatment for cancer. That accounts for my unprofessional conduct."

ABOUT A YEAR LATER, Limpert gave an interview to *The Washington Journalism Review*. He talked about the many excuses writers use for failing to produce a printable article. One of his eleven amusing stories was called "The Keep Your Mouth Shut Lesson."

Limpert said: "A long-overdue piece arrives. Too long and wanders all over the place. Writer says he knows it's not any good but he figures I can help him rewrite it. All the frustrations of the past year come out and I really lay into the guy, tell him I'm tired of people expecting me to do what any self-respecting professional writer ought to do before he brings a piece in. He is shaken, but takes it. I feel better. The next day I get a letter from him saying by the way, the reason it took him so long to finish the piece is that he's got cancer and the radiation therapy has been very hard on him."

DURING MY CANCER TREATMENT, my body was beyond my control, as was my ability to think clearly and improve my emotional state. I'd always been impatient and impulsive, and I refused to accept my limitations. Had I not fought so hard—especially against depression—the experience would have been easier.

If I'd been wise, I'd have accepted with grace and resignation the fact that my life was going to get worse before it got better. Instead of inflicting pride and fear of humiliation on others, I could have recognized that nothing was going to reduce the time required for cancer therapy.

I expected too much of myself, constantly berating myself, feeling ashamed of my body and my emotions. I needed to acknowledge that I was sick, and sick people often do not behave well. I pushed myself to do things I was incapable of doing. When I failed, I luxuriated in self-pity and remorse. My intolerance and contempt for my own behavior made everything more difficult.

19

DAVID IS MY CLOSEST FRIEND. We became room-mates after I ran off to San Francisco in 1972 during the painful period following the breakup of my marriage. I am angry that David is so far away.

YEARS LATER, David described his initial reaction to my cancer. "When you told me about it, I felt as if a huge clang had sounded, like a steel door dropping shut, separating us. There was no way I could participate in what you were going through. It was as if someone had driven a wedge into our friendship."

MY LETTERS to David attempt to overcome the sense of isolation. "Without any apparent order," I write, "I've been reading about my disease. There is, for example, a medical journal called *Cancer*. It's on the same shelf as *Chest*, *Lungs*, and—my favorite—*Pain Magazine*.

"I've been trying to figure my odds, which is difficult. The American Cancer Society gives a 70–80 percent chance of the cancer not killing me within the next five years—even higher odds if you include dying but not dead. HEW says that Hodgkin's disease patients in my category have a better than 50 percent survival rate for fifteen years. That assumes that their categories are analogous to the ones used on me. There are even thirty- and forty-year survival rates. But none of these statistics is specifically applicable to me. The odds are probably much better for my form of treatment, which, however, is too new to have accurate statistics.

"Considering the 'miracles of modern science,' it does seem likely that I will outlive this disease. Still, it's sobering (if that's the right word) to realize that I will never know for certain whether my cancer has been cured. If I get hit by a truck and die at ninety-five, have they cured me of cancer? *They* don't know. Of course, an autopsy might tell, but by then it's a bit late.

"Death waits for each of us. Considering everything, death is likely to take a different form for me than Hodgkin's disease. Still, I think about me and the disease constantly, feel it especially strong every day at eleven when I see my fellow cancer patients and wonder what they've got and how long they'll live."

THE FIRST ROUND of treatment ends on Thursday, July 22. Dr. Diem examines me.

"What happens next?" I ask.

"You go to your primary physician, Dr. Falk, for an

examination. We give you about four weeks for your body to recover. Then you'll be exposed to another round."

Although I am afraid of the answer, I ask, "Will I have to undergo chemotherapy?"

"No. I don't think so. You seem to be responding well. But that's a decision your physician has to make. Why, did he say he wanted to give you chemotherapy?"

"He said he'd first see how I responded to radiation treatments before deciding."

"Well," Dr. Diem says, committing himself more strongly than usual, "you seem to be responding quite well, and I don't see any reason for it. But that's up to your physician to decide."

"What about a third round of therapy at my pelvis?"

"I don't think that'll be necessary. The results of your spleen and liver biopsy don't indicate that it's necessary. At this point, I see no purpose in extending the field of treatment."

Chemotherapy has become a major fear. Others in the basement waiting room have experienced it, telling me that radiation is mild by comparison. After a while, I literally shudder when I even think about chemotherapy—shaking slightly, feeling weak around the knees, experiencing a cold wave of panic that something could be worse than this.

Before my appointment with Aaron the following week, I prepare arguments over why I'll refuse if he orders chemotherapy. Dr. Diem's information is another item added to my list. If necessary, I promise myself, I'll change doctors. Or I'll let the cancer kill me.

When Aaron examines me, I timidly raise the subject, afraid of mentioning it for fear of invoking the deed.

Aaron cavalierly dismisses it. "Why, did I say something about chemotherapy?"

"Yes. You said you'd decide depending on how I responded to radiation."

"Oh yes, I remember saying that. But you're doing really well. Didn't I tell you that chemotherapy will be unnecessary?"

"No."

"Well, you're doing so well. I just wanted to keep it as an option. But I should have told you I dismissed it."

"Yes," I say, "you should have. Will the next round of treatment really be the end?"

"Yes."

Aaron explains the reason for the next round of radiation. "Standard radiation technique historically confined itself to the immediate site. Accordingly, your treatment would be over now. However, patients who are also irradiated at the next level down—at the next grouping of lymph nodes [where the cancer would probably spread next]—were found to have better survival rates.

"So your next round of treatment is for prophylactic reasons. We want to make sure we get it all. Fortunately the operation results confirmed that your Hodgkin's disease has not spread to your abdomen. Otherwise a third round of treatment at your pelvic area would be necessary."

AARON was playing it safe. The lymphangiogram (the test where they slit open my feet) showed dark spots at the base of my lungs. Although the subsequent operation found no presence of disease and although medical evidence favors tissue samples over other kinds of tests, Aaron worried that there was a slight possibility that the lymphangiogram might be correct.

On that off chance, he wanted to monitor me closely, reserving the option of additional radiation treatments and even, if necessary, chemotherapy. Since no tumors appeared and my blood and chest X rays continued to be clean, Aaron now felt safe in concluding that the next round of radiation should end my cancer treatment. Because pelvic irradiation increases the risk of genetic damage and sterility, his decision helped keep open my option to become a parent.

In part Aaron was being careful because he had been embarrassed by the original misdiagnosis. Being careful is part of Aaron's nature, and he wasn't going to make a major decision about my care without checking and double checking. Certainly, his caution caused me to worry—perhaps, unnecessarily. But would I have wanted a doctor who was less careful?

EVEN AFTER the treatments stop, I feel worse as my body reacts to the cumulative dose. It takes about two weeks before the downward cycle of exhaustion and depression reverses. On Sunday August 8, 1976, Laura and I awaken early. I am cranky. I can't decide whether to stay in bed or leave it. All summer long I've talked about going for a boat ride on the Potomac. Laura says, "Why don't we do that?" Going seems less effort than deciding. I reluctantly agree.

We leave my apartment at about ten. The dock is near the Lincoln Memorial. Crossing the Mall to the boat, we pass the Smithsonian Institution's Folk Life Festival—a cross between a circus and a country fair. There are tents and people riding horses, climbing poles, and singing German folk songs. I feel some of the crowd's excitement and say, "If I feel up to it after the boat trip, maybe we can walk around the fair." Laura says skeptically, "We'll see." This is my first real outing since the hospital, and my willingness even to go on a boat ride is unusual.

The ride is marvelous. It is one of those hot noisy crowded tourist boats that has no destination and just cruises a few miles on the river before returning to the pier. Yet, somehow, I feel better just being outside, seeing the lush Virginia shore, Washington's impressive monuments, planes taking off from National Airport, birds circling the river. By the end of the ride I am excited and enthusiastic. This is my first burst of energy in months. The difference between feeling half dead and feeling alive is intensely noticeable. I had forgotten what being alive really feels like. I don't want to stop experiencing this marvelous phenomenon.

The festival is sprawled out across the Mall for nearly a dozen blocks. One booth features handicrafts from Alaska. An artisan is manufacturing a dogsled. I have never been to Alaska or on a dogsled and the idea of doing both suddenly intrigues me. I ask lots of detailed questions: "What kind of wood do you use?" "How did you get into the dogsled business?" "How fast does a dogsled go?"

Then we walk to a country music concert, look at show horses and farm animals, watch a greased-pole-climbing contest and a fire-rescue demonstration. I don't want to return to the car until dark, and only agree to postpone looking at the sunset from the water's edge and then, maybe, the stars, when Laura says she is tired.

It never occurs to me that Laura would get tired. I am the one who always complains of exhaustion. We must have walked three or four miles that day, but I'm not tired.

Laura observes, "You obviously got a spurt of energy. We walked around the entire folk festival at least nine times, and we watched every display there was. It was fun, but it was like trying to cram three weeks into one day. It was exhausting, but it didn't exhaust you. You kept right on going."

Now that I have my energy back, I try to make up for lost time. However, the newly regained energy is not constant. Some days I am fine. On others I fade early or am unable to get started. The variations bring abrupt shifts in mood. I get panicky when it becomes apparent that the time available to concentrate on and complete a task is limited and not dependable.

I do realize that this recovery period is not going to last, that I will be subjected to a second round of radiation. Unlike the last round, this time I prepare.

My major concern is how I am likely to be affected by the radiation, which will be directed at my belly. The first round was made considerably worse by my being surprised by predictable side effects. This time I plan to avoid being caught off-guard. I don't want to ask Aaron about likely side effects, because he'll just tell me to ask Dr. Grey. If he is even available, Grey will give me a runaround, and the other radiologists will be guarded and evasive. Also, until I absolutely have to, I don't want to return to that basement.

My friend Andy reminds me that his father is a radiologist. "He prides himself that he is unlike most radiologists who are more comfortable with their machines than with their patients. Here's his phone number. Call him at home."

Andy coaches me. "Tell him that this is an informal request. Stress that you're not dissatisfied with your current physician, but you simply want information about likely side effects. Say that you realize that any information he gives will be general in nature and may not apply to your specific condition."

Dr. Schwartzman explains that because treatment will be directed toward my midsection, my liver will get "a good share of radiation." This may cause loss of appetite and nausea. The intestinal tract itself, he says, frequently becomes "sensitive" and "upset," adding to the nausea and probably causing diarrhea.

The information reassures me. Now that I know how my body is likely to react, I can focus on other concerns.

I decide to boil down my cancer experience into two and a half typewritten, dispassionate pages for the Op-Ed section of *The New York Times*. After all, I tell myself, when I put something down on paper I understand it better. Also I tend not to believe things until I see them in print. I figure that if *The Times* says I'm not going to die, then I can believe *The Times*—even if I am doing the writing.

Describing my anger at having cancer is painful. Describing the radiation treatment is awful. Describing why I'm going to live is guilt-provoking—it causes me to think about those who won't live. On balance, however, analyzing my lack of control helps me accept it.

Once I have written the article, I have difficulty over my original decision to publish it. True, I've already used cancer to escape criminal prosecution and evade professional responsibility. Even so, I can hide my disease so it need not become common knowledge in my professional and—except for intimates—personal life. After all, I've made a modest reputation writing about agricultural policy. Do I want to endanger that reputation by publicizing something as intensely personal as cancer? What will disclosure do to my career possibilities? Even though I say I will live, if people read I have cancer, won't they automatically assume I'm going to die?

On the other hand there is the danger, given my psychological background, that if I keep my cancer a secret it will assume a power of its own. Like my grandfather's non-Jewishness, the family will discuss it only in whispers and guard it from outsiders.

Indeed, this kind of secrecy does not suit my personality. I do not want to spend my life putting energy into hiding my secret. After all, based on reliable statistics I have an excellent chance of surviving without the cancer affecting either my lifespan or my life-style. But already part of me believes that having cancer is something to be ashamed of. Throughout the month of July, I've been reading and rereading the book of Job—brooding about the relationship between God and disease. My cancer often makes me feel humiliated. If I can be open about it, I can rob the disease of some of its power over me.

I mail the article, having decided that while to some degree the reaction of others to my cancer is my problem, primarily it is theirs. On balance I decide the advantages of disclosure much outweigh the disadvantages.

My career needs attention. I recognize the importance of planning beyond treatment, of having something to do when October arrives and my cancer becomes history. I am afraid that if I don't repair and maintain professional contacts there's a danger that the cancer experience will assume more importance than it actually has. Come October, I want to be busy. I don't want to brood over what I might have done if only the cancer experience hadn't happened.

I make an appointment with Marty Peretz, owner of *The New Republic*. The magazine publishes my articles, and its book company is scheduled to publish my agriculture book. Although Marty and I get along well and my articles have been well received, the lateness of my book is straining our relationship.

I tell Marty that the delay is partially due to my Hodgkin's disease treatment, which is nearly over, and that Joan Tapper, my book editor, and I are meeting tomorrow to develop a schedule for completion of the manuscript.

Marty says that a close friend had Hodgkin's disease. "The doctors told him it would kill him. He outlived their predictions and is fine. He even was able to have children."

"Children? He was able to have children?"

"He was concerned about genetic damage," Marty says, "but apparently, it wasn't a problem. His children are bright and healthy. . . ."

This information cheers me enormously. I feel as if I too can live a normal life. Also, Marty agrees to release part of the advance money on the book. That will alleviate some of my financial pressures.

The business lunch with Joan Tapper is useful. "Perhaps when you finish the agriculture book," she says, "you might write one about your cancer experience."

The idea terrifies me. "I'm not ready to write that book. All I want to do is finish this one."

Taking out my red Leathersmith notebook, I rattle off chapters that need to be written and provide due dates. The next day I mail her a memo and a new timetable.

Meanwhile Washington is caught up in the excitement of the election campaign. A jubilant Democratic convention in

New York has just nominated a man who seems almost certain to win. Washington, which is basically a Democratic town, is suddenly alive with men and women—some of whom are friends—who have ambitious plans for getting prestigious jobs in the new administration. I don't expect the election to bring the millennium, but as a Democrat from birth, I believe Carter's election will be good for the country and suspect that it might even be personally good for me.

Like any reporter, I want to write about the election. In the course of keeping current I call Republican headquarters the day after their convention and ask for a copy of the platform. Even though the platform fight was a front-page squabble, headquarters doesn't have a copy and I am given a runaround. This amuses me, and I tell David Sanford, managing editor of *The New Republic*, that the Republican party is unable to locate a copy of its own platform. "Write it up."

The platform article's publication cheers me. I have the feeling that I am being a reporter again. I get enormous pleasure out of seeing my name in print. It proves to me that I am still alive and working, someone whose career has survived cancer and radiation.

Then I mail Joan Tapper the next chapter earlier than scheduled. I meet with Jack Limpert at the *The Washingtonian*. He agrees to my revision plan, and I send him the article. I also write articles for *The New Republic*, about embargoing food—which has suddenly become a campaign issue—and about Earl Butz's forced resignation as secretary of agriculture.

Despite these developments, I recognize that I need a steady income. I need a job. I begin looking seriously, applying for a consultancy with an energy research firm, an editorial job for the National Association of Housing and Redevelopment Officials, and a writing job in rural Pennsylvania for Rodale Press, which publishes literature on growing organic food.

I am delighted when Rodale Press decides to pay for a trip to Pennsylvania. I haven't been out of Washington for months. Driving a rented car through the beautiful Pennsylvania countryside is pure joy. Emmaus is a quiet, pretty town. I enjoy visiting Rodale Press's editorial offices, looking at the research farm and the experiments in raising catfish.

At lunch I drink Scotch and smoke an unfiltered Camel cigarette. This is the first time in months that I enjoy eating again and get pleasure from drinking liquor and smoking. I know these pleasures will soon be wiped out by the next round of radiation. So, I indulge them with gusto, probably too much gusto considering that I am at the center of the organic health industry.

The job would pay well. When I return from the trip, an hour before Karen's eighth birthday party, I tell Laura about the interview. She is outraged that I flaunted my "vices."

"You don't want the job anyway," she says.

"Sure I want the job. But I don't want them thinking I'm someone I'm not. They're hiring a writer. If they're too up tight to deal with the fact that I smoke and drink, then they shouldn't hire me. If I move up to Emmaus, Pennsylvania, and you and the kids come with me, I want to make sure that my job will be secure enough to accommodate my personal habits."

Neither of us is convinced, and we remain angry with each other.

"I have no idea what the fuck is happening with Laura and me," I write David. "I've never been as intimate with anyone. We love each other. I can even say how the love works and why we're good for each other. True, I'm crazy, but she's crazy, too. Ever since the divorce, there has been the obvious opportunity for us to live together and get married and each of us is scared shitless. Sometimes I think the laundry list of my misdeeds toward her is so large that it can never be overcome. Nothing is ever forgotten. It sits there like a historical marker waiting to be read at the next round of battle."

In the past, I've been able to penetrate Laura's protective screen of anger and shyness (a curious combination). She'd tell me that she was afraid to express negative feelings, concerned that aggression would frighten me into withdrawal. When I was well, I was often able to reassure her, to let her know that her honesty was appreciated, that although it might frighten me, my fear was less important than the honesty necessary to keeping us together.

I decide that my cancer has made communication difficult and I schedule an appointment for us both to see Paul. At first Laura is reluctant to describe her anger. Then she lets it out. "I'm sick of you taking me for granted. I'm tired of hearing you complaining and whining. You know, you insensitive prick, I have problems of my own."

I tell her how much I care for her, how much her help means to me. "Sometimes I feel that whatever I do, you'll regard what I give you as too little, too late."

"Try me," she says. "You make a lot of demands, you are difficult to be with, and you aren't very much fun."

THE RADIATION treatments resume. I get a new set of purple dye lines—rectangles on my belly and back. The waiting room is predictably depressing, but less so. I know I am going to be done soon. One morning, when Trudie is sliding my body under the linear accelerator, she tells me—yet again—"If I had to pick a disease to have, I'd pick yours." Instead of snarling at her, I believe her.

Each Friday I check off another week in my Leathersmith notebook. The nausea is not as bad as expected. Dr. Wilson, a staff radiologist who is too consistently optimistic, gives me gray pills—Phenegran. They don't really help, but I don't much care.

The diarrhea is not as bad as I feared. Lomotil—a little white pill that Dr. Wilson prescribes—works instantly. Fellow patients tell embarrassing stories about being unable to control their bowel movements. I am spared that.

Every Thursday, I grow increasingly concerned about my blood tests and weight. I don't want anything to stop the treatments and postpone the end. So I am especially diligent about forcing food into my system. I don't concentrate only on calories, but even try to eat nutritious foods.

I am getting used to sudden losses of energy. Ritalin soon stops having any effect. I reread Tom Wicker's *Facing the Lions*, all the Nero Wolfe mysteries, Ross Thomas, Irwin Shaw, Gore Vidal, and the Travis McGee books. Sometimes, as with *Tinker, Tailor, Soldier, Spy*, I reread the book as soon as I finish it. I grow more adept at dealing with the boredom that comes when the energy disappears. Toward the end I just watch television day and night, sliding off into oblivion with a badly needed sleeping pill. I am often too tired to sleep.

Laura's patience with me is exhausted. She gets short-tempered about my taking so many pills—a small white pill for energy, a smaller white pill for diarrhea, a gray pill for nausea.

She snaps at me. "What do you need all that for? Are you running a pharmacy?"

At first, I put considerable effort into trying to please her and spending time with the children. When I am too weak, I promise that soon I'll be better and we can settle down to a life together. When the radiation sickness is at its worst, I don't seem to need her as much. I don't feel as dependent or grabby. I talk about us and our future together, but it makes her nervous. Something unsettling has happened to us, to the way we relate to each other.

On September 22, a Wednesday, my cancer treatment ends. Dr. Toller examines me. Of the four available doctors, Toller is my favorite. I'm sorry I didn't meet him earlier. He is reassuringly dour. When I ask, he tells me the worst possible consequences of my disease and treatment. It is a form of honesty I am grateful for. He tells me that I am fine. "Come back in a month for a routine exam. You should also see Dr. Falk for a wrap-up exam."

Except for physicals every six months—blood tests, chest X rays, feeling for lumps at my neck, arms, and groin—I am done with cancer and its treatment. Done!

I ask, "Is there any reason why I shouldn't have children?"

"What do you mean?"

"Well, I think Dr. Grey said that I shouldn't propagate any children for at least several months after radiation for genetic reasons."

"That doesn't sound right," Toller says. "He couldn't have meant that. The beam is highly concentrated, and any scatter should be out of your testicles and your system immediately, as soon as the machine is turned off. You don't need to be concerned about genetic damage. The statistical variation is negligible." * He pauses. "That means your chances of having healthy children are about as good as anyone else's. However, if I were you, I wouldn't have any children for a year and a half to two years."

"Why?" I ask.

"Well, if I were you, I'd want to know that I'd be alive to see my children grow up. The chances are that if the Hodgkin's disease doesn't come back within a year and a half or two years, you'll survive."

"I thought the American Cancer Society definition for cure is five years."

"That's an approximate figure for all forms of cancer. Some cancers are longer than five years. Some are shorter. With Hodgkin's disease, a year and a half to two years is a more precise figure. If you have a relapse, your odds drop sharply. If you survive two years without symptoms, chances are high that it won't come back. If I were you, I'd wait two years before having children. That way you will know whether you'll live."

---

* Both Dr. Grey and Dr. Toller [not their real names] were correct. Although the concentrated beam was directed elsewhere, a relatively slight portion of the beam (scatter) reached the testicles. As soon as the machine was turned off, no radiation was left in the body. However, has the slight dose of radiation that hit the testicles increased the risk of a genetically deformed child if I immediately father a child? Some radiologists, like Dr. Toller, argue that the risk is negligible. Others, like Dr. Grey, suggest that it is prudent to wait about six months so that all sperm that may have been genetically affected by the scattered radiation are replaced. Specialists are engaged in a lively debate on the subject which is discussed in the medical literature. Reader-patients who are considering fatherhood should consult their physician.

20

O N TUESDAY, April 5, 1977, I awaken early. It is nearly a year since I was told I had cancer. I phone the neighborhood pharmacy and ask for delivery of a bottle of sleeping pills, five hundred aspirin, and a six-pack of Coke. When the package arrives, I put the sodas on the side of the bed. I empty out the medicine cabinet, throwing drug bottles onto my blanket. I carefully get into bed and count the stash. I have forty-two Dalmane, twenty-two Percodan, and forty Valium. Will that kill me or should I take two hundred aspirin? Or both? I decide the aspirin will be unnecessary. I swallow handfuls of sleeping pills, pain pills, and Valium and wait to die.

I turn on the telephone answering machine, then I write out a will, leaving everything to Laura.

I write, "To whom it may concern: I changed my mind. There were too many things to do, and I felt I couldn't finish any of them. I found myself standing at the end of an old life and the beginning of a new life, and I wanted the new life, but felt too sick, too dispirited to handle it. I didn't want to live and be a failure. I don't have the energy to be a success. It seems to me that death will provide another opportunity. There is some place where I am going to, and maybe there I can better appreciate the sanctity of life, of my life."

Before the drugs take effect, I get up to drink Scotch. I bring the bottle and glass back to bed and begin sipping, waiting.

During the next few days I am in a foglike stupor. At some point I am cold and turn on the space heater. The blanket catches in the heater, but I don't realize that it is on fire until I feel my left heel burning. I throw Coke on the flames, which puts out the fire. I return to sleep or whatever that drugged state is.

When I awaken I am surprised that I failed to kill myself. Rather than try again, and succeed, I decide that once is enough. I feel miserable. The dope in my system makes it difficult to focus. My mouth is really dry, and I am hungry. My burnt heel makes getting up painful. Under my door someone has slipped a telegram: "Attempts to reach you by phone unsuccessful. Concerned about your welfare." It is from Paul.

PAUL ASKS ME to describe the attempted suicide to group. I don't want to, but do. I see that there's shock—or is it fear?—throughout the room.

Sally says, "After all that . . ."

Jack gives one of his long rambling analyses. He uses the words *accident*, *infancy*, *help*.

I don't want to hear what anyone is saying. I find myself surprised that these people care about me.

Paul is angry. He says, "Of course you had to use my prescriptions. Thanks a lot." His tone changes. "I suspected that you might try something like this." I can hear the affection in his voice. "Of course, I didn't know when it would come. You intended to fail, didn't you?"

"I don't think so," I say slowly, confused by the suggestion. I know that some use suicide as a way of getting attention, but I'm not one of those people. At least, I don't think I am.

"It was an act of independence," Paul continues. "You had to prove to yourself that you are free to kill yourself. If you are free to die, you are free to live. You're making progress."

Lois enters the room late. "Joel just tried to kill himself," Paul says. The news bulletin startles her. It also startles me. I realize that trying to kill myself was—for want of a better word—significant.

"Why did you do it?" she asks.

"I don't know," I answer automatically, trying to avoid examining what I've done.

IT MAY BE USEFUL to describe the events that proceeded my suicide attempt.

On October 12, 1976, I turn 29. Now that radiation is over, I want to blot that period of my life out of my memory. I want to forget doctors, pain, and discomfort as quickly as possible. I do not want to consider the possibility of a relapse. My birthday comes weeks after my last exposure to the linear accelerator. I don't want to waste time thinking about how grateful I am to be alive. I have a living to earn and a life to straighten out.

I don't know why I asked Toller about children. I am certainly not interested in having any. After all, Laura has three, and having a child is the last thing either of us needs. Perhaps I have a macho desire to be reassured that cancer and its treatment has not somehow robbed me of my "manhood"— whatever that is.

After radiation ends, Laura is impatient for me to fulfill my promises. She took care of me for so long. "Now it's my turn," she says. I promised that things would get better. However, just like after the first round of radiation, I feel worse after this round. After the cumulative dose catches up with me, it takes almost two weeks before the cycle reverses. Then, because my resistance is so low, I get the flu. After the flu, I continue to feel weak and not quite healthy. My body needs time to recover fully and to replace the dead cells. The recovery is not difficult. I even begin riding my bicycle again, but my stamina is not what it was. It takes about six months until I feel normal—the way I did before the cancer experience.

Gradually, Laura and I begin to go out more frequently, to restaurants, parties, and on trips to the country. I go to her house more often. I do things with the kids, like taking Luke to the Inaugural Parade. However, I feel that the more I do with Laura and for her, the more she tells me it isn't enough. By February I feel overwhelmed. I can never make up to her for all she has done for me. I am perpetually in her debt. I am always reminded that nothing can ever erase it.

I love her. I realize that when you love someone the way I love Laura the love will always remain. The sex continues to be intense and passionate, somehow immune from contamination. However, when we talk about anything—politics, the weather, her work, my work, our attitudes about the world—it always leads to a fight. I feel as if I am forever on the losing side of whatever the argument happens to be. Our arguments take place wherever we happen to be—even in public places, something I find excruciatingly embarrassing. All too often, she yells at me in a crowded restaurant.

In February I say, "I can't take it anymore. I think we should stop seeing each other."

"I agree," she quickly replies. "I've had enough of this. It's a good idea for us to split up before we completely destroy the good feelings we have for each other."

I am disappointed that she agrees so readily. Did I want her to change my mind?

Life without Laura is lonely. At the end of each day, I grow acutely aware of how much I miss her, pacing up and down my narrow messy apartment, realizing that she is not expected. I walk impatiently to the Capitol and sit on the steps. As I watch the sun set over Washington, I feel sad that Laura isn't here to share this with me.

I mope like an adolescent, uninterested in other women. Often I want to call Laura. I rehearse excuses that might justify casual conversation. Just as often I stay home rather than go out, staring at the phone, hoping it will ring and she'll be on the other end. Why, I ask myself, did I bother to get cured if I can't have Laura?

I AM FEELING overwhelmed and at times frightened by my new job as a consultant to the Congressional Office of Technology Assessment (OTA). I am writing a report on a USDA-administered program called WIC (Women, Infants, and Children). OTA's Food Group is sponsoring a conference, paying more than a dozen experts to fly to Washington to discuss WIC and the health and nutritional problems of pregnant women. In three years the Food Group has published only one report. In order to justify (among other things) the expense of the conference, a report is needed quickly. The Food Group immediately pushes through my hiring in time for me to cover the conference.

The job quickly turns into a major undertaking. The conference participants don't understand what is expected of them and cannot agree on what WIC is supposed to do. Eventually I learn that the experts' confusion is primarily caused by the confused state of the program.

There is uncertainty about whether WIC is a food program or a health program, even though it was created as an experiment to improve the health of pregnant women. Its statutory objectives are to feed the poor, reduce infant mortality, and promote nutritional education simply by giving each recipient $22 a month worth of such items as eggs, breakfast cereal, infant formula, juice, milk, and cheese. However, administrative costs are high. If WIC's purpose is to feed the poor, there are less expensive ways of providing them with even more food. If its purpose is to reduce infant mortality, it makes more sense to establish or improve medical facilities rather than rely on iron-fortified Total or Kaboom cereal to reduce anemia in pregnant women. If its purpose is nutritional education, there are better methods than ordering pregnant women not to share omelets with their children.

By the time I realize what I have gotten into, I am in way over my head. Although in four years WIC has grown from a $20 million "experiment" into a $200 million program, USDA does not have even basic records on how many people are receiving benefits and where. The report I'm writing requires a staff, computer, and budget—none of which is available. However, my report might be the closest thing to an official evaluation.

After several months of work, I become convinced that WIC should be scrapped and replaced with a major effort to reduce infant mortality. But WIC has an effective constituency of nurses, nutritionists, and poverty activists. They admit that WIC has "faults." They are afraid that a budget-conscious Carter Administration—if given the excuse—will kill the program rather than replace it with an alternative.

The report is already hundreds of pages long, but I am unwilling to finish and take responsibility for the country's unborn children. It frightens me that I might be responsible for killing a program that is feeding indigent pregnant women. What right do I have to deny others life and health? I become obsessive about this. I start dwelling on my own mothering and my own nutrition. How can I write this? What if I'm wrong?

MY CAREER generally is not going well. In September my friend David Sanford, managing editor of *The New Republic*, is induced by a big salary increase to take a job in California. In October Marty Peretz rejects two of my articles that Sanford commissioned. His curt rejection note suggests that I finish my book before submitting more articles.

The Washingtonian doesn't like the rewrite of the agriculture department article, and Limpert suggests that I give up the effort. I finish the first draft of my agriculture book by March 1, but Joan Tapper and I both agree that a rewrite is necessary. I have an interview to become the speechwriter for the secretary of commerce. After I submit a sample speech Juanita Kreps decides to hire someone else.

There are occasional good developments. I convince Marty to make an exception to his ban, and he publishes a piece describing the operations of Cargill, a multinational grain trading company. The consulting work at OTA pays enough to support me, which is a welcome change.

But I want more than I am getting. I want a secure and prestigious career. Instead I am facing overdue deadlines and unhappy editors. Each success is temporary and is followed by several failures. I feel as if my career is getting progressively worse, with no relief in sight and no way of avoiding some ill-defined but inevitable disaster. I am discouraged.

IN NOVEMBER, the Op-Ed page of the *Times* surprises me by publishing my article on cancer. Reading in November what I wrote in July, I feel like a stranger following someone else's story. I don't want to think about cancer. I am sorry that I have written about it.

The *Times* entitles the piece "A New Lease on Life." That certainly isn't the way I feel. The article reads, "Slowly, I have come to understand that life has been given to me for a second time." Instead, I feel that the effort was a waste of time and money—that life, whether on the first try or the second, is too much work for too little reward.

The reaction to the article surprises me. Nothing I've written before has ever produced this kind of response. Without consciously intending to, I have touched my readers in a surprisingly profound way. I have done some good by writing about my cancer experience.

Suddenly strangers are telling me about their cancer treatment. They say that my article has given them hope, that finally someone is describing what they experienced, someone who had cancer and doesn't equate it with death. I have made fellow cancer patients feel less alone at a time when public perceptions about cancer are still in the Dark Ages. (The American Cancer Society's most recent Conference on Human Values and Cancer was still obsessed with that bullshit question: Is it a good idea to tell the patient he has cancer?)

A woman from Minnesota, who was cured of Hodgkin's disease, tells me that she knew of no one else who had not died from it. She says that it makes her feel less frightened to know there is someone out there she can write to, someone alive. A lawyer from New Jersey says that he has been through a similar experience, that he has "resumed normal living" but knows no one else who has been successfully treated. A friend of a friend, who read the article, is due for a six-month checkup. She also had Hodgkin's disease and has apparently been cured, but she is afraid the tumors will come back. Although they haven't returned, she is frightened. She has never talked to anyone about her fear of cancer. She talks to me, she says, because I've survived treatment and understand.

I am afraid of dealing with the responsibility. The letters and calls make it seem as if I know something my fellow patients don't. I feel empty inside, like a depressed hypocrite talking about how precious life is.

I receive a second set of responses from my family. My father suddenly calls from Florida. "Are you all right?" he asks, concerned. After a relative sent him a copy of the article, he was suddenly taking seriously in November what had been serious back in May. For over six months, we've communicated through phone calls and perfunctory letters, and throughout he has had trouble even remembering the name of my disease. "That organ they took out . . . ?" he asks.

"You mean my spleen?"

"Yes, your spleen. Do you need it?"

"No, I don't need it," I tell him and laugh.

He tells me how worried he is, and I calm him down. After the conversation, I am angry. *Where the hell were you when I needed you?*

A cousin, whom I have not seen in years, sends a certified check for a hundred dollars. My grandmother phones. She's very upset. "Why did you have to write about it?" For my family, the *Times* article has made me an instant celebrity. As numerous long-distance calls and cards testify, I will now and forever be "the cancer patient"—someone who is asked "How are you?" in a tone that is noticeably different.

By March, I get enough money together to take a long weekend in Florida. I don't tell my parents about the breakup with Laura. I want to show my father and mother that I am all right. Last time Mother saw me was in the hospital, still connected to tubes. Now I am swimming in the condominium pool.

Mother has become withdrawn and depressed. The closeness that used to exist between us has been replaced by awkwardness. For the past few months, Mother has been working on a novel, a thinly veiled autobiographical account. Our telephone conversations have been increasingly dominated by progress reports on the novel and requests for advice. Now, when she isn't talking about novel-writing technique, she talks about wanting to explain herself. She doesn't want to explain herself now, however, but rather at some future date, when the book is published. "It will be a legacy," she says. "Then, you'll truly understand me." Although our old relationship is over, a new one has not really emerged. She realizes this and reacts to her feelings of pain by talking about her need to explain and be understood.

Meanwhile, my father wants to be reassured that I'm all right. "It's a very confusing illness," he says. "Like so many people, I didn't expect that it could happen to my immediate family. I know very little about it, very little about cancer." He says that he isn't motivated to find out more. "I don't want to know about it. I skip articles about cancer. I'm not interested. If I had some medical training, I might have been motivated, but it is so beyond me. I regard it as a highly tragic situation, but I don't know what to do about it."

I tell him about the biopsy, the results of the exploratory operation, the purpose of radiation treatment, and how the odds mean that I am likely to live. He seems unable to grasp the information. I see from the way he looks at me that he's worried and that no matter what I say, he cannot be reassured. My seventy-five-year-old father is convinced that his son is going to die.

WHEN I RETURN from Florida, my wound infection acts up again. A stitch bubbles to the surface of my belly, bringing redness and pus. In his office, Simpson cuts out the stitch and looks around for more. After a month of nightly baths—washing out the pus and waiting for the damn thing to heal—I go back to Simpson's office. He finds another stitch and suggests that if it doesn't clear up, I go back to the hospital for outpatient surgery. "The light's better there," he explains. We do that. He finds three more stitches, and I spend an uncomfortable weekend bathing my wound and popping pain pills. It flares up again and in his office he removes yet another suture.

This process terrifies me. Although my belly has healed,

finally, I worry that I will have to go back continually for more cutting and probing. My body disgusts me. When the infection flares I become nauseated by the smell of pus. I frequently examine my scars in the mirror, worrying about how noticeable they are, afraid that no woman could ever love someone who looks as mutilated as I feel.

FOR YEARS, I continued to hold on to the idea that I wanted to kill myself but failed simply because I didn't know enough about dose levels. However, I knew at the time that if I took all that aspirin I would be dead. Using suicide as a way of expressing despair and asking for help is pathetic as well as bad melodrama. Clearly, if I wanted to tell Laura I was angry I had healthier ways of doing so than by making her the beneficiary of my handwritten will (when I had nothing to leave). The danger in suicide attempts, of course, is miscalculation. I may have wanted to fail, but if I had popped enough pills, drunk enough Scotch, or failed to put out the fire, I would have succeeded anyway. The whole incident does not reflect well on me and my behavior, to say the least.

Analyzing the ingredients for an effective suicide is not the point. I tried to kill myself despite the fact that I knew I'd survived cancer. I did it because the strain of accepting the disease, going through treatment, and resuming a "normal life" was too much. The events that led up to the attempt illustrate my frame of mind. I was vulnerable to suicide, my emotions were overloaded, and I reached a breaking point.

Paul later observed, "There's a kind of depression that tends to occur in cancer patients that seems to be biological, that seems to be part of the cancer. But this is different. There is a subgroup of cancer patients who 'solve depression' through their cancer. For instance, during the year after the loss of a mate, the onset of cancer in the husband or wife is far more frequent than would be expected from the statistical tables. The spouse 'solves' the loss by turning it into a malignant tumor.

"Keep in mind that reality is multioriented. Psychoanalytic thinking treats reality in one way; biological thinking treats it another way. But they're describing the same element."

Biological thinking holds that no one knows what causes Hodgkin's disease. The suspicion is that it is caused by a virus. A study in *The New England Journal of Medicine* entitled "Childhood Social Environment and Hodgkin's Disease" observes that incidence of Hodgkin's disease is higher among patients who are Jewish, come from small families, and have mothers who are well-educated and protective during early childhood.

Concerning psychoanalytic thinking, Paul said, "When infants are deprived of mother's love, they go into a serious depression and turn to the wall. Because of a failure of primary separation between mother and child, some people remain vulnerable to that kind of face-to-the-wall depression for part or all of their lives.

"Before your cancer, the work you and I were doing was depriving you of your 'mother,' " Paul said. "In that setting you were very vulnerable to depression and, as a matter of fact, were somewhat depressed on the basis of that separation. In such a case, it's well known that some people develop tumors. The tumor is one response in some people to this kind of loss. And the mechanism is rage, rage at the loss. The rage is internalized. Internalized anger is depression. And a tumor is an internal way of denoting anger. In the tumor is rage mixed with—kind of larded with—love. This was your rage at the bond that had lasted into your maturity. When you were forced to give up that bond, it formed into a tumor. The tumor—the cancer—was one last stand, as it were.

"Now that last stand was taken from you." As a result, Paul observed, after I was cured of cancer, "You were lonely without it." The suicide attempt was one last try at solving depression by being self-destructive. Having failed, it became clear that I could live without being dependent or depressed. I was liberated from the bond that had tied me to an immature form of behavior. I was now free to have what Paul chooses to call "a viable adulthood."

IT IS SEPTEMBER 1981, and Diana and I will be married in a month. The details seem never-ending—mailing out invitations, having the rings inscribed, not looking at her dress during the fittings, renting a gray cutaway with striped pants, writing the wedding service. During a pause between errands I ask Diana, "Do you understand Paul's theory that my having cancer was a way of holding on to Mother?"

"No."

"Even if you realize that Mother is not my mother as she is today, but my inability—back in infancy—to develop an independent personality?"

"No, it sounds too complicated. I don't understand it, and I don't think anyone else will, either. It sounds strange."

I say, "I don't want people to think I'm crazy."

"No matter how you present it," she says, "people don't regard seeing a psychiatrist as normal." Diana was born and raised in the Midwest. I assume she possesses an innate ability to discern how "healthy" mainstream Americans react. "People assume they can solve their own problems, that if you need help there's something wrong with you."

"What about my suicide attempt? Do you understand why I tried to kill myself?"

"Yes. You were feeling dejected. You went through a hard time, and it caused you to be discouraged. It was enough to discourage anyone."

21

THE CANCER ITSELF left little effect upon my body. It did take about six months for all my hair to grow back. The new hair has a slightly different texture—it is softer and finer, but the difference is only noticeable to the touch. My wound infection finally cleared up, and my scars are now healed and faded. The combination of radiation and loss of spleen made me slightly more susceptible to bacterial infection. I was immunized against that risk by a one-time-only vaccine.

About two years after the final round of radiation, a small lump appeared at my groin. I worried about it. Aaron said it was probably nothing. (Lumps at the groin are less likely to be cancerous than those under the arm or at the base of the neck.) When the lump did not go away, Aaron suggested that Simpson remove it. As Aaron, Simpson, and even I expected, it was not cancerous.

For the first few years I had routine medical examinations

every six months. Now I go once a year. The examination takes twenty minutes at most. It consists of a chest X ray, some blood tests, and Aaron rubbing my nodal areas with his fingers to check for lumps. It is painless, and Aaron and I both are bored by it. My cancer treatment happened more than five years ago, and no future treatment will be necessary. I have never taken cancer drugs and none will be necessary. My physical activity is not limited in any way as a result of cancer and its treatment. Aaron says, "By all odds, now greater than 95 percent, you're cured forever. The Hodgkin's disease is dead."

I continued in group until Paul and I decided that I was ready to "graduate." On my last day, we had a small wine-and-cheese party. Everyone sat on the floor, reminiscing about the changes we had made. Doris said that she admired my courage in dealing with the cancer experience.

I still miss the twice-weekly group sessions and the feeling of family that evolved. I miss Jack's ability to synthesize actions into coherent theory. I miss Lois's crisp, no-nonsense approach to emotions. I miss Doris's warmth and directness. I miss Sally and our brother-sister rivalry and closeness. I miss Paul and his skill at guiding me. Most of all, I have the bittersweet feeling that comes from being unable to regularly share joy with those with whom I regularly shared sorrow.

Paul said, "Having cancer was the best thing that ever happened to you." He was right. Conquering the disease helped me to conquer my fear of death. Surviving the panic that followed—like a delayed time bomb—helped me survive my fear of life.

Paul once described the "correct" emotional response to the cancer experience as "I am who I am." The patient recog-

234

nizes that he is not exactly the same as a result of confronting the issue of death and will always be more aware of the malfunctions of his body. He defines that understanding in the expression: "I'm still okay, even though the balances have shifted a bit."

Today Mother and I relate to each other as adults, something I never thought possible. As my father observed, "Not only have you changed, but people around you have changed, like your mother and myself. We accept the fact that you have been through a great tragic business, that you've suffered—you've suffered enough—and we're more responsive to the things you have to say and the things you do."

Despite frequent attempts, Laura and I were never able to reestablish our relationship. We had reconciliations which sometimes were so intense and wonderful that it seemed impossible to believe that we could ever be apart. For one glorious week, we vacationed in Nassau, making love on powder-white beaches, drinking champagne in the tropical moonlight, and making future plans to conform with our honeymoonlike setting. Somehow the plans never seemed to work out. The anger, guilt, and expectations that surfaced during the cancer experience always returned. After a while the reconciliations became shorter and the periods between them longer. Today, we're friends. A sadness remains that despite our love for each other, we were unable to establish a life together.

I finally did finish the study on the WIC program. I rewrote the agriculture book. I became a full-time consultant to Congress's General Accounting Office, rewriting reports to make them more interesting and comprehensible. The experience at GAO helped establish a new pattern for my career.

Not only was I earning a living, but I also seemed to acquire a confidence in my job skills that I hadn't had before. I was able to meet deadlines, and I even learned how to work within a bureaucracy.

Then I landed a prestigious job as a political appointee in the labor department, working for the under secretary, writing speeches and dealing with press policy. Although my bosses and fellow employees at GAO were sorry to see me go, they were pleased about my new opportunity. The job pressures at the labor department were frequently intense, but there too I did well. Today, in a changed Washington, I've even learned to write Republican speeches.

I met Diana at the labor department. We met while I was writing a speech on the Multifiber Arrangement for the importation of textiles. She is an expert on the subject. After our first few dates, I told her about the Hodgkin's disease. She reacted to the information like one listening to a veteran who had survived a bad war. She was sympathetic that I once had a hard time, but did not see how it affected our relationship. We love each other. For each of us, our love helps make the future a goal worth reaching.

Before getting married, I suggested to Diana that we talk to Aaron about my Hodgkin's disease. Aaron was thrilled that we were consulting him. He reassured Diana that I am cured.

I wanted him to discuss two possible consequences of my treatment. First, the medical literature points to increased incidence of leukemia in Hodgkin's disease survivors. "The increased incidence of leukemia," he said, "is primarily in those patients who've been treated with chemotherapy plus total nodal radiotherapy. You did not have chemotherapy and you did not have total nodal. [Total nodal includes the pelvic area. My radiation only reached down to the area around my belly.] So, although your chance of getting leukemia is probably higher than mine, it's not the increased incidence that's bandied about in the literature. Perhaps the marginal increase would put you at one point two cases per one hundred thousand rather than one case per hundred thousand. I don't think that's significant."

Then I wanted to know about considerations regarding children. He said, "Your genitalia were not radiated. The chances are your fertility is normal."

"So the likelihood of genetic defects is the same as for the rest of the population?"

"The chances are you incurred no gonadal chromosomal damage because you were shielded during radiation. Probably the risk of genetic defects is a little bit higher than the rest of the population. There are figures on chemotherapy plus total nodal radiation, but again you had neither. I don't think I could get a figure on the incidence of birth defects for your form of treatment. It's probably marginally higher than the rest of the population, but not enough to stop from having children—if you want children. Do you want children?"

"Yes," I said. "Probably."

"Oh, how nice," Aaron said enthusiastically. "Really? God, you're really getting serious, aren't you?"

"I'm getting married."

"I know, but you're getting serious about all of life— having children and everything. I think that's great. I would push right ahead."

Diana laughed. "Not so fast. One thing at a time."

"I mean," Aaron said, "from the point of view of whether or not your history should constrain you in any way, the answer is no. It shouldn't. Absolutely not."

I asked, "You are, of course, coming to the wedding?"

"I wouldn't miss it for the world," Aaron said.

As I started Diana's yellow Karmann Ghia, she turned to me. "Not only were you cured of cancer, but you're not limited or affected by it in any way. You were incredibly lucky."

ACKNOWLEDGMENTS

For saving my life, I thank the real Aaron Falk, for his timely work in identifying my cancer, causing it to be cured, generally making sure that I am here today, and putting up with my constant questions and my ever-present tape recorder. Also, I thank the real Cory Simpson, who cut out my cancer; the pathologists, who went through the Eureka process, everyone in George Washington University Hospital's Division of Radiation Oncology and Biophysics, whose success at destroying my cancer has made it possible for me to bitch about the magazines in the waiting room; and George Washington University Hospital as an institution—including its many physicians, students, nurses, orderlies, janitors, and administrators—because its bureaucratic regulations and the people who establish and enforce them (at all levels) ensure that medicine does work (and also because it helped me in the research on this book). Although I have never met them, I also thank

Henry S. Kaplan, the Medical Establishment's Hodgkin's disease guru, whose research and radiation techniques made it possible for others to save my life; and Vincent T. Devita of the National Cancer Institute, who was instrumental in developing cures for advanced stages of Hodgkin's disease.

For special assistance in a category by itself, I thank Paul S. Weisberg, not only for telling me, at a timely moment, that I would live, but also for teaching me how to enjoy life. I thank Jack Raher, for whom fondness grows each year; the group, as a body and individually, because sometimes a family can be established without relatives; and James Masterson, for describing the tie and teaching how to break it.

For being there when I was sick, I thank the real Laura Constable. She taught me how to love, and she had the courage, years later, to discuss into a tape recorder her recollections and feelings about my cancer experience and our unrealized hopes. I thank Laura's children and family. I thank my mother, whose love for me has always been consistent, even when I was unable to accept it. I thank my father, Isadore. David F. Phillips, Andrew Jay Schwartzman, and John Lee Avery have each given me friendship, which will last as long as we do. I thank Frances Collin, my agent, who inherited the tradition of grace and quality the late Marie Rodell established and who has made that tradition her own; Fran gave me great hope before I was sick, when I was sick, and after I recovered, and she is the midwife to this book and, I trust, many others. I also thank my grandmother, Alvin and Theresa Demick, *Arts Magazine,* Norman and Phyllis Demick, Miriam Daniel, William Gahr, Jack Brock, the Community and Economic Development Division of GAO, Deborah Matz, the Food Group of the Office of Technology Assessment, David

Sanford, Martin Peretz, Joan Tapper, Gwen Somers, *The New Republic*, Jack Limpert of *The Washingtonian*, Diana McLellan (The Ear), Hubert Humphrey, Earl Butz, Cesar Chavez, Phillip Moery, Patric Mullen, Eileen Shanahan, Michael Andrews, Walter Shapiro, Donald Dunnington, Agnes Mravcak, Dorothy Row, Susan Dankoff, Lynne Murphy, sugar, Joel Schwartzman, Howard Bray, the Fund for Investigative Journalism, the Hay-Adams Hotel, rice, Susan Herskowitz, Washington Independent Writers, the commodity-futures markets, Blue Cross/Blue Shield, Jack Halpert, Louis and Ida Solkoff, Ben and Lil Solkoff, and Ed Sacks. I am also grateful for the written word of Ross Thomas, Gore Vidal, Eric Ambler, Dick Francis, John le Carré, Irwin Shaw, Rex Stout, and God for keeping me company and the *I Ching* for, among other things, warning: "The caution of a fox walking over ice is proverbial. ... A young fox who as yet has not acquired this caution goes ahead boldly, and it may happen that he falls in and gets his tail wet when he is almost across the water. Then of course his effort has been all in vain."

For helping to create this book, I thank Donald Hutter, who knew what I wanted to say before I even did and without whom this would not be a book; Wendy Moonan, who at *The New York Times Magazine* believed I had something to say; David Schneiderman, who caused my first cancer account to be published on the Op-Ed page of the *Times*; Richard W. Seaver, my publisher at Holt, Rinehart and Winston, who demonstrated his faith; Paul Bresnick, my editor; and Robin Mayers, who not only typed and retyped the manuscript, but also improved my thinking and writing.

For aid and comfort, I thank my wife Diana, whom I love intensely, for her love and encouragement (even when I was working on this book and metaphorically kicking the cat) and for her faith in our future. I thank Sarah, my mother's second only child, who is a continual source of joy. I thank Diana's cat Zookie, who still doesn't understand what I do. I thank the District of Columbia Public Library and its director Hardy R. Franklin, the Library of Congress, National Library of Medicine, National Cancer Institute, American Cancer Society and Lois Nelson Callahan of its Washington chapter, and The Candlelighters Foundation for the hope and skills it gives to the children who survive cancer. I also thank Linda Lazarus, the Media Access Project, Betty Hood, Josephine Bass, Robert Bass, Lillian Fuller, Robert J. Brown, Craig Berrington, the U.S. Department of Labor, Andrew L. Rothman, the Securities and Exchange Commission, Edwin H. Friedman, the late Frederic M. Vogelsang, the National Association of Housing and Redevelopment officials, my grandmother's friend Bess, *Changing Times* magazine, Barbara Machtiger, the Foreign Policy Study Foundation, Paul Boertlein, Robin Schollmeyer, Jack Skigen, the National Press Club, National Public Radio, the Capitol of the United States, Paul Schwartzman, and Klaudia (a friend from a previous decade who always bought books by living writers—rather than take them out of the library—"because they need the royalties"). And I thank the late John Wayne, who told me that two months after his initial treatment for cancer he was making a movie: "I dove into a river with handcuffs on in January . . . and that was tough. It kept me from developing a protection which I thought I needed but which I didn't need. The thing to do is just try your damndest without telling anyone else about it." As this book proves, I couldn't follow his advice, but I respect it.